Mediterranean Diet Cookbook

---

188 Easy, Flavorful & Healthy Mediterranean Recipes to Lose Weight and Reset Your Metabolism

Erika Davidson

Table of Contents

Introduction **9**

The Mediterranean Diet Pyramid 10

Benefits of the Mediterranean Diet 14

Chapter 1: Breakfast **18**

Cheesy Olives Bread 18

Sweet Potato Tart 19

Hummus and Tomato Breakfast Pittas 20

Baked Ricotta & Pears 21

Egg White Scramble with Cherry Tomatoes & Spinach 22

Blueberry, Hazelnut, and Lemon Breakfast Grain Salad 23

Feta Frittata 24

Fruit Bulgur Breakfast Bowls 25

Tuna Sandwich 26

Yogurt Figs Mix 27

Mango and Spinach Bowls 27

Oregano Quinoa and Spinach Muffins 28

Apricots Couscous 29

Tapioca Pudding 30

Banana and Quinoa Casserole 30

Spiced Chickpeas Bowls 31

Avocado Spread 32

Greek Beans Tortillas 33

Ham & Egg Cups 34

Spinach and Artichoke Frittata 35

Avocado and Egg Breakfast Pizza 36

Spinach Feta Breakfast Wraps 37

Summer Vegetables with Eggs 38

Crispy White Beans with Greens and Poached Egg 39

Caprese Avocado Toast 40

Huevos Rancheros..41

Marinara Eggs With Parsley - Gluten-Free....................................42

Nutty Orange Polenta..43

Feta & Quinoa Egg Muffins...44

5-Minute Heirloom Tomato & Cucumber Toast.............................45

Garbanzo Bean Salad 46

Brown Rice Salad..47

Tahini Pine Nuts Toast...47

Feta - Avocado & Mashed Chickpea Toast.....................................48

Stuffed Pita Breads..49

Blueberries Quinoa...50

Endives, Fennel and Orange Salad...50

Raspberries and Yogurt Smoothie..51

Homemade Muesli 51

Tangerine and Pomegranate Breakfast Fruit Salad 53

Chapter 2: Side Dishes 55

Bulgur, Kale and Cheese Mix...55

Spicy Green Beans Mix 56

Beans and Rice 56

Lime Cucumber Mix..57

Walnuts Cucumber Mix 58

Cheesy Beet Salad..58

Rosemary Beets 59

Squash and Tomatoes Mix..60

Balsamic Eggplant Mix 61

Sage Barley Mix 61

Chickpeas and Beets Mix 62

Creamy Sweet Potatoes Mix...63

Cabbage and Mushrooms Mix...64

Lemon Mushroom Rice..64

Paprika and Chives Potatoes 65

Lemony Carrots 66

Tomato and Millet Mix 67

Quinoa and Greens Salad 68

Veggies and Avocado Dressing 68

Cauliflower Quinoa 69

Mixed Veggies and Chard 70

Spicy Broccoli and Almonds 71

Balsamic Asparagus 72

Chapter 3: Lunch **73**

Avocado & Tuna Tapas 73

Greek Baked Zucchini & Potatoes 73

Chickpeas Soup 74

Tomato Soup 75

Oyster Stew 76

Potatoes and Lentils Stew 77

Chicken Salad..78

Chicken Skillet 79

Green Beans & Feta 81

Kale - Mediterranean-Style 81

Mediterranean Endive Boats 82

Salmon With Warm Tomato-Olive Salad..83

Shrimp & Penne..84

Tilapia With Avocado & Red Onion 85

Berries and Grilled Calamari 86

Cajun Garlic Shrimp Noodle Bowl... 88

Tarragon Cod Fillets 89

Salmon and Radish Mix 89

Smoked Salmon and Watercress Salad 90

Salmon and Corn Salad 91

Mediterranean Nachos 92

Mediterranean Potatoes 92

Turkey Fritters and Sauce 93

Stuffed Eggplants 94

Delicious Roasted Duck 96

Duck Breast with Apricot Sauce 97

Mediterranean Duck Breast Salad 98

Duck and Orange Sauce 99

Duck Breast and Blackberries Mix 101

Slow Cooked Mediterranean Duck 102

Salmon Bowls 103

Spicy Potato Salad 104

Chicken and Rice Soup 105

Fish Soup 106

Lamb and Potatoes Stew 107

Ground Pork and Tomatoes Soup 108

Melitzanes Imam/Greek Eggplant Dish 109

Red Mediterranean Potato Salad 110

Savory Mediterranean Orzo 111

Spinach Pie 112

Cannellini Bean Lettuce Wraps 113

Easy Farfalle with Fresh Tomatoes 114

Fried Rice With Spinach - Peppers & Artichokes 115

Gigantes (Greek Lima Beans) 116

Gluten-Free Spanish Rice 117

Chapter 4: Dinner 119

Spaghetti in Clam Sauce 119

Creamy Fish Gratin 120

Broccoli Pesto Spaghetti 120

Spaghetti all'Olio 121

Quick Tomato Spaghetti 122

Creamy Chicken Soup 123

Barley and Chicken Soup...124

Chili Oregano Baked Cheese 125

Braised Chicken & Artichoke Hearts 126

Chicken Thighs With Shallots In Red Wine Vinegar 127

Feta Chicken Burgers...128

Grecian Chicken & Pasta Skillet..129

Greek Penne & Chicken 131

Easy and Simple Chicken 132

Dill Relish on White Sea Bass 133

Fish and Orzo 134

Baked Sea Bass..135

Fish and Tomato Sauce 135

Halibut and Quinoa Mix..136

Lemon and Dates Barramundi...137

Fish Cakes 138

Baked Salmon With Dill 139

Couscous With Pepperoncini & Tuna..140

Herb-Crusted Halibut..141

Pan Roasted Chicken and Potatoes 142

Crispy Italian Chicken 143

Sea Bass in a Pocket 144

Chicken and Chorizo Casserole...144

Lamb Stuffed Tomatoes with Herbs 145

Creamy Spinach with Polenta and Poached Egg..............................146

Grilled Vegetable Feta Tart 148

Tomato and Halloumi Platter 149

Chickpeas and Millet Stew 150

Chapter 5: Snacks **152**

Traditional Mediterranean Hummus..152

Tuna Salad in Lettuce Cups...152

Rice Burgers 153

Wheatberry Burgers 154

Easy Nachos...155

Eggplant Bites...156

Peanut Butter Yogurt Dip 157

Roasted Chickpeas 158

Salty Almonds..159

Cheesy Artichoke Dip..159

Date and Fig Smoothie.. 160

Cucumber Bites with Creamy Avocado 161

Tomato Finger Sandwich 161

Parsley Cheese Balls 162

Layered Dip...163

Grilled Tempeh Sticks 164

Sweet Potato Fries 164

Italian Style Potato Fries...165

Lemon Cauliflower Florets 166

Chapter 6: Desserts...168

Poached Cherries... 168

Watermelon-Strawberry Rosewater Yogurt Panna Cotta.................... 169

Mascarpone and Ricotta Stuffed Dates 170

Glazed Mediterranean Puffy Fig... 171

Figs Pie...172

Cherry Cream...173

Strawberries Cream...174

Apples and Plum Cake 174

Cinnamon Chickpeas Cookies 175

Cocoa Brownies 176

Cranberries and Pears Pie..177

Lemon Cream 178

Blueberries Stew...178

Mandarin Cream 179

Creamy Mint Strawberry Mix 179

Vanilla Cake 180

Pumpkin Cream 181

Grapes Stew.. 182

Cocoa Sweet Cherry Cream 182

Apple Couscous Pudding.. 183

Ricotta Ramekins... 184

Papaya Cream 184

Mediterranean Stuffed Custard Pancakes... 185

Mediterranean Cheesecake 187

Mediterranean Bread Pudding 188

Banana Shake Bowls.. 190

Mediterranean Biscotti... 190

Chocolate Baklava... 192

Orange-Glazed Fruit and Ouzo Whipped Cream............................... 194

Conclusion..196

Introduction

The Mediterranean diet refers to the traditional eating habits and lifestyles of the people living around the Mediterranean Sea – Italy, Spain, France, Greece, and some North African countries. The Mediterranean diet has become very popular in recent times, as people from these regions are known to have better health and suffer from fewer ailments, such as cancer and cardiovascular issues. Food plays a key role in this.

Research has uncovered the many benefits of this diet. According to the results of a 2013 study, many overweight and diabetic patients showed a surprising improvement in their cardiovascular health after eating the Mediterranean diet for 5 years. The study was conducted among 7,000 people in Spain. There was a marked 30% reduction in cardiovascular disease in the high-risk group.

The report took the world by storm after the New England Journal of Medicine published the findings. Several studies have indicated its many health benefits as well. The Mediterranean diet may stabilize blood sugar, prevent Alzheimer's disease, reduce the risk of heart disease and stroke, improve brain health, ease anxiety and depression, promote weight loss, and even lower the risk of certain types of cancer.

The diet differs from country to country and even within the regions of these countries because of cultural, ethnic, agricultural, religious, and economic values. So there is no one standard Mediterranean diet. However, there are several common factors.

The Mediterranean Diet Pyramid

The diet's food pyramid is a nutrition guide to help people eat the right foods in the correct quantities at the prescribed frequency as per the traditional eating habits of people from the Mediterranean coast countries. The pyramid was developed by the World Health Organization, Harvard. The Mediterranean diet food pyramid is easy to understand. It provides an easy way to follow the eating plan.

The Food Layers

1. Whole grains, pieces of bread, beans – The lowest and the widest layer of foods are strongly recommended. Your meals should be made mostly of these items. Eat whole-wheat bread, whole-wheat pita, whole-grain rolls, whole-grain cereal, whole-wheat pasta, and brown rice. 4 to 6 servings a day will give you plenty of nutrition.

2. Fruits and vegetables – This is almost as important as the lowest layer. Eat non-starchy vegetables daily like asparagus, broccoli, beets, tomatoes, carrots, cucumber, cabbage, cauliflower, turnips at 4 to 8 servings daily. Take 2 to 4 servings of fruits every day. Choose seasonal fresh fruits.

3. Olive oil – Cook your meals preferably in extra-virgin olive oil. Make it a daily consumption as it is healthy for the body, lowers low-density lipoprotein cholesterol (LDL) and total cholesterol level. Up to 2 tablespoons of olive oil is allowed. The diet also allows canola oil.

4. Fish – Now, we come to the food layers that are to be consumed weekly and not daily. You can have fish 2 to 3 times a week. Best is fatty sea fish like tuna, herring, salmon, and sardines. Sea fish will give you heart-healthy omega-3 fatty acids and plenty of proteins. Shellfish, including mussels, oysters, shrimp, and clams, are also good.

5. Poultry, cheese, yogurt – The diet should include cheese, yogurt, eggs, chicken, and other poultry products, but in moderation. Maximum 2-3 times in a week. Low-fat dairy is best. Soy milk, cheese, or yogurt is better.

6. Meats and sweets – This is the topmost layer consisting of foods best avoided. You can have them once or twice a month max. Remember, the Mediterranean diet is plant-based. There is very little room for meat, especially red meat. If you cannot live without it, then eat red meat in small portions. Choose lean cuts. Have sweets only to celebrate. For instance, you can have a couple of sweets after following the diet for a month.

Recap of Recommended Foods

Most people living in the region eat a diet rich in whole grains, vegetables, fruits, nuts, seeds, fish, fats, and legumes. It is not a restrictive diet like the many low-fat eating plans. Actually, fat is encouraged, but only from healthy sources, such as polyunsaturated fat (omega-3 fatty acids) that you will get from fish and monounsaturated fat from olive oil.

The diet is strongly plant-based but not exclusively vegetarian. It recommends limiting the intake of saturated fats and trans fats from red meat and processed foods. You must also limit the intake of dairy products.

· Fruits and vegetables – Eat these daily. Try to have 7-10 servings every day. Meals are strongly based on plant-based foods. Eat fresh fruits and vegetables. Pick from any seasonal varieties.

· Whole grains – Eat whole-grain cereal, bread, and pasta. All parts of whole grains – the germ, bran, and endosperm – provide healthy nutrients. These nutrients are lost when the grain is refined into white flour.

· Healthy fats only – Avoid butter for cooking. Switch to olive oil. Dip your bread in flavored olive oil instead of applying margarine or butter on bread. Trans fats and saturated fats can cause heart disease.

· Fish – Fish is encouraged. Eat fatty fish like herring, mackerel, albacore tuna, sardines, lake trout, and salmon. Fatty fish will give you plenty of healthy omega-3 fatty acids that reduce inflammations. Omega-3 fatty acids also reduced blood clotting, decreased triglycerides, and improves heart health. Eat fresh seafood two times a week. Avoid deep-fried fish; rather, choose grilled fish.

· Legumes – These provides the body with minerals, protein, complex carbohydrates, polyunsaturated fatty acids, and fiber. Eat them daily.

· Dairy and poultry – You can eat eggs, milk products, and chicken throughout the week, but in moderation. Restrict cheese. Go for plain or low-fat Greek yogurt instead.

· Nuts and seeds – 3 or more servings every week is perfect. Eat a variety of nuts, seeds, and beans. Walnuts and almonds are all allowed.

· Red meat – The Mediterranean diet is not meat-based. You can still have red meat, but only once or twice a week max. If you love red meat, make sure that it is lean. Eat only small portions. Avoid processed meats like salami, sausage, and bologna.

· Olive oil – This the diet's key source of fat. Olive oil will give you monounsaturated fat that lowers the LDL or low-density lipoprotein cholesterol and total cholesterol level. Seeds and nuts will also provide monounsaturated fat. You can also have some canola oil but no cream, butter, mayonnaise, or margarine. Use up to 4 tablespoons of olive oil a day. For best results, only take extra-virgin olive oil.

· Wine – Red wine is allowed but in moderation. Don't drink more than a glass of red wine daily. Best take only 3-4 days a week.

· Desserts – Say no to ice cream, sweets, pies, and chocolate cake. Fresh fruits are a good alternative with natural sweetness.

Main Components of the Diet at a Glance

· Focus on natural foods – Avoid processed foods as much as you can.

· Be flexible – Plan to have a variety of foods.

· Consume fruits, vegetables, healthy fats, and whole grains daily.

· Have weekly plans for poultry, fish, eggs, and beans.

· Enjoy dairy products moderately.

· Limit red meat intake.

· Drink water instead of soda. Only drink wine when having a meal.

Benefits of the Mediterranean Diet

We've also heard about the Mediterranean diet's advantages. It helps fight obesity and provides for cardiovascular health for which it has been called one of the best known diets.

Our modern lifestyle is quicker than ever and with less time to devote not only to the kitchen but also to ourselves, causing us to eat inappropriately and with excessive amounts of fats and chemical components that impact our health.

The Mediterranean diet means a diverse and balanced combination of natural and conventional items from a beautiful region bathed by the Mediterranean Sea that enjoys a particular lifestyle. Fruits, fruits, legumes, cereals, olive oil as a source of fat, fish, and eggs, and poultry are essential in more moderate amounts.

The Mediterranean diet, as the Mediterranean Diet Foundation site says, is a significant cultural heritage that is much more than just a nutritious, rich, and balanced template. Will you know the benefits of dieting à la Mediterranean? Continue reading. We will tell you everything about it!

The importance of this diet has made it recognized by the United Nations Educational, Scientific and Cultural Organization (UNESCO) as an Intangible Heritage of Mankind. It also has a traditional and customary character because it includes cultural and folkloric influences.

It advises eating foods involving both the use of healthy ingredients and healthy preparation methods. Because of its inherent characteristics, it is not only a high-flavored diet but it is also rich in benefits for our health.

Benefits of the Mediterranean Diet

1. Fight the so-called bad cholesterol

The abundant consumption of seafood, fish, and vegetables, as opposed to the moderate intake of red meat, is one of the main benefits of the Mediterranean diet. This is linked to a decrease in indices of cholesterol.

2. It is beneficial for the heart

Due to the presence of unsaturated fatty acids in combination with nitrates and dietary nitrates, the Mediterranean diet helps to reduce the risk of cardiovascular diseases. Nuts, fish oil, olives, and avocado contain such valuable fatty acids.

3. It prevents stroke

Strokes are one of the most common clinical conditions today. Anything we can do to limit them is welcome.

The Mediterranean diet significantly reduces the risk of suffering a stroke as it is rich in olive oil and nuts. This is in line with the findings of the Center for Human Nutrition and Aging Research at Tufts University in the US and the researchers at the Carlos III Health Institute.

4. Avoids stomach problems

Combined with polyphenols (antioxidant substances) in apples and red wine, green vegetable nitrates function as a gastric defender. They avoid stomach problems such as ulcers and help to alleviate them if you have them already.

5. Controls diabetes

Thanks to a low-fat diet and unsweetened desserts, the Mediterranean diet helps control type 2 diabetes.

6. Decreases the risk of Alzheimer's and dementia

In the Mediterranean diet, eggs are an important element. Due to the optimum state of the blood vessels that result, this food improves brain functions. Hence, the risk of mental deterioration in people following this diet is decreasing.

7. Helps against obesity

Adequate healthy food intake, reasonable carbohydrate and fat consumption, as well as the inclusion of vegetables and fruits, and certain proteins enables both weight loss and ideal weight maintenance.

8. Help prevent Parkinson's disease

The foods on this diet have great antioxidant power, which prevents cell deterioration and reduces the chance of suffering from Parkinson's disease.

9. Protects the bones

Adequate intake of calcium-rich products helps to strengthen the bones, which in turn helps prevent fractures and bone conditions.

10. Provides agility

The nutritious foods from this diet favor muscle firmness and muscle, which means more physical fitness, regardless of age.

11. Anti-aging

The abundance of antioxidants and calcium, as well as the reduced likelihood of suffering from different conditions, suggest better physical health and, with it, a healthy, long, and productive life.

Chapter 1:
Breakfast

Cheesy Olive Bread

Preparation Time: 1 hour and 40 minutes

Cooking Time: 30 minutes

Servings: 10

Ingredients:

4 cups whole-wheat flour

3 tablespoons oregano, chopped

2 teaspoons dry yeast

¼ cup olive oil

1 and ½ cups black olives, pitted and sliced

1 cup water

½ cup feta cheese, crumbled

Directions:

- In a bowl, mix the flour with the water, yeast, and oil; stir and knead the dough well.
- Put the dough in a bowl, cover with plastic wrap and keep in a warm place for 1 hour.
- Divide the dough into 2 bowls and stretch each ball well.
- Add the rest of the ingredients to each ball tucking them inside, and knead the dough again.
- Flatten the balls a bit and leave aside for 40 minutes.
- Transfer the balls to a baking sheet lined with parchment paper, make a small slit in each, and bake at 425 degrees F for 30 minutes.

- Serve as a Mediterranean breakfast.

Nutrition: calories 251, fat 7.3, fiber 2.1, carbs 39.7, protein 6.7

Sweet Potato Tart

Preparation Time: 10 minutes

Cooking Time: 1 hour and 10 minutes

Servings: 8

Ingredients:

2 pounds sweet potatoes, peeled and cubed

¼ cup olive oil+ a drizzle

7 ounces feta cheese, crumbled

1 yellow onion, chopped

2 eggs, whisked

¼ cup almond milk

1 tablespoon herbs de Provence

pinch of salt and black pepper

6 phyllo dough sheets

1 tablespoon parmesan, grated

Directions:

- In a bowl, combine the potatoes with half the oil, the salt and pepper. Toss and spread on a baking sheet lined with parchment paper, and roast at 400 degrees F for 25 minutes.

- Meanwhile, Heat a pan with half the remaining oil over medium heat; add the onion and sauté for 5 minutes.

- In a bowl, combine the eggs with the milk, feta, herbs, salt, pepper, onion, sweet potatoes, and the rest of the oil and toss.

- Arrange the phyllo sheets in a tart pan and brush with a drizzle of oil.

- Add the sweet potato mix and spread it into the pan.

- Sprinkle the parmesan on top and bake covered with tin foil at 350 degrees F for 20 minutes.

- Remove the tin foil, bake the tart for 20 minutes more, cool it down, slice, and serve for breakfast.

Nutrition: calories 476, fat 16.8, fiber 10.2, carbs 68.8, protein 13.9

Hummus and Tomato Breakfast Pittas

Preparation Time: 5 minutes

Cooking Time: 10 minutes

Servings: 4

Ingredients

4 large eggs, at room temperature

salt, to taste

2 whole-wheat pita pieces of bread with pockets, cut in half

1/2 cup hummus

1 medium cucumber, thinly sliced into rounds

2 medium tomatoes, large dice

handful of fresh parsley leaves, coarsely chopped

freshly ground black pepper

hot sauce (optional)

Directions:

- Take a large saucepan, fill with water, and place over medium heat until it boils.

- Add the eggs and cook for 7 minutes.

- Immediately drain the water and place the eggs under cool water until they cool down. Set to one side until you can handle them comfortably.

- Peel the eggs and cut into 1/4" slices, sprinkle with salt, and set to one side.

- Take a pita pocket and spread with hummus, fill with cucumber and tomato, season well, then add an egg.

- Sprinkle with parsley and hot sauce; serve and enjoy.

Nutrition: Calories: 377 Net carbs: 17g Fat: 31g Protein: 11g

Baked Ricotta & Pears

Preparation Time: 15 minutes

Cooking Time: 30 minutes

Servings: 4

Ingredients:

White whole wheat flour (.25 cup)

sugar (1 tbsp.)

nutmeg (.25 tsp.)

ricotta cheese - whole-milk (16 oz. container)

large eggs (2)

diced pear (1)

water (2 tbsp.)

vanilla extract (1 tsp.)

honey (1 tbsp.)

Also needed: 4 - 6 oz. ramekins

Directions:

- Warm the oven to 400° Fahrenheit.

- Lightly spritz the ramekins with cooking oil.

- Whisk the flour, nutmeg, sugar, vanilla, eggs, and ricotta together in a large mixing bowl.

- Spoon the mixture into the dishes. Bake for 20 to 25 minutes or until they're firm and set. Transfer them to the countertop and wait for them to cool.

- In a saucepan, at medium heat, toss the cored and diced pear into the water for about ten minutes until slightly softened.

- Take the pan from the burner and stir in the honey.

- Serve the ricotta ramekins with the warm pear when ready.

Nutrition: Calories: 312 Protein: 17 grams Fat: 17 grams

Egg White Scramble with Cherry Tomatoes & Spinach

Preparation Time: 5 minutes

Cooking Time: 8-10 minutes

Servings: 4

Ingredients:

olive oil (1 tbsp.)

eggs (1 whole) & egg whites (10)

black pepper (.25 tsp.)

salt (.5 tsp.)

minced garlic clove (1)

halved cherry tomatoes (2 cups)

packed fresh baby spinach (2 cups)

light cream or half & half (.5 cup)

finely grated parmesan cheese (.25 cup)

Directions:

- Whisk the eggs, pepper, salt, and milk.

- Prepare a skillet at med-high heat.

- Toss in the garlic when the pan is hot and sauté for approximately 30 seconds.

- Pour in the tomatoes and spinach and continue to sauté for one additional minute. The tomatoes should be softened and the spinach wilted.

- Add the egg mixture into the pan using the medium heat setting. Fold the egg gently as it cooks for about two to three minutes.

- Remove from the burner and sprinkle with a sprinkle of cheese.

Nutrition: Calories: 142 Protein: 15 grams Fat: 2 grams

Blueberry, Hazelnut, and Lemon Breakfast Grain Salad

Preparation Time: 5 minutes

Cooking Time: 10 minutes

Servings: 8

Ingredients

1 cup steel-cut oats

1 cup dry golden quinoa

1/2 cup dry millet

3 tablespoons olive oil, divided

¾ teaspoon salt

1 x 1" piece fresh ginger, peeled and cut into coins

2 large lemons, zest, and juice

1/2 cup maple syrup

1 cup Greek yogurt

1/4 teaspoon nutmeg

2 cups hazelnuts, roughly chopped and toasted

2 cups blueberries or mixed berries

4 1/2 cups water

Directions:

- Take a mesh strainer and add the oats, quinoa, and millet. Wash well, then set to one side.

- Find a 3-quart saucepan, add a tablespoon of the oil, and place over medium heat.

- Add the grains and cook for 2-3 minutes to toast.

- Pour in the water, salt, ginger coins, and lemon zest.

- Bring to the boil, then cover and turn down the heat. Let simmer for 20 minutes.

- Turn off the heat and let sit for five minutes.

- Fluff with a fork, remove the ginger, then cool for at least an hour.

- Take a large bowl and add in the grains.

- Take a medium bowl and add the remaining olive oil, lemon juice, maple syrup, yogurt, and nutmeg. Whisk well to combine.

- Pour this over the grains and stir well.

- Add the hazelnuts and blueberries, stir again, then pop into the fridge overnight.

- Serve and enjoy.

Nutrition: Calories: 363Net carbs: 60g Fat: 11g Protein: 7g

Feta Frittata

Preparation Time: 15 minutes

Cooking Time: 25 minutes

Servings: 2

Ingredients:

garlic (1 small clove)

green onion (1)

large eggs (2)

egg substitute (.5 cup)

crumbled feta cheese - divided (4 tbsp.)

plum tomato (.33 cup)

avocado slices (4 thin)

reduced-fat sour cream (2 tbsp.)

Also needed: 6-inch skillet

Directions:

- Thinly slice/mince the onion, garlic, and tomato. Peel the avocado before slicing.

- Heat the pan using the medium temperature setting and spritz with cooking oil.

- Whisk the egg substitute, eggs, and three tablespoons of the feta cheese.

- Add the egg mixture to the pan. Cover and simmer for four to six minutes.

- Sprinkle with the rest of the feta cheese and tomato. Cover and continue cooking until the eggs are set about two to three more minutes.

- Wait about five minutes before cutting it into halves.

- Serve with avocado and sour cream.

Nutrition: Protein: 17 grams Fat: 12 grams Calories: 203

Fruit Bulgur Breakfast Bowls

Preparation Time: 15 minutes

Cooking Time: 20 minutes

Servings: 6

Ingredients:

2% milk (2 cups)

uncooked bulgur wheat (1.5 cups)

water (1 cup)

cinnamon (.5 tsp.)

frozen/fresh pitted dark sweet cherries (2 cups)

dried/fresh chopped figs (8)

chopped almonds (.5 cup)

Directions:

- Combine cinnamon, water, milk, and bulgur.
- Stir once and bring to a boil. Cover the pot. Reduce the temperature setting to medium-low.
- Continue cooking until the liquid is absorbed (approx. 10 min.).
- Extinguish the flame or heat, but leave the pan on the stove and stir in the cherries (frozen or thawed), almonds, and figs.
- Stir well to thaw the cherries and hydrate the figs. Stir in the mint, and scoop into servings bowls.
- Serve with warm milk, or serve chilled to your liking.

Nutrition: Protein: 9 grams Fat: 6 grams Calories: 301

Tuna Sandwich

Preparation Time: 5 minutes

Cooking Time: 0 minutes

Servings: 2

Ingredients:

6 ounces canned tuna, drained and flaked

1 avocado, peeled, pitted, and mashed

4 whole-wheat bread slices

pinch of salt and black pepper

1 cup baby spinach

1 tablespoon feta cheese, crumbled

Directions:

- In a bowl, mix the tuna with the cheese, salt, and pepper and stir well.

- Spread the mashed avocado on the bread slices, divide the tuna mix among 2 of them, divide the spinach as well, top with the other 2 slices, and serve for breakfast.

Nutrition: calories 283, fat 11.2, fiber 3.4, carbs 9.8, protein 4.5

Yogurt Figs Mix

Preparation Time: 5 minutes

Cooking Time: 5 minutes

Servings: 4

Ingredients:

8 ounces figs, chopped

2 cups Greek yogurt

1 tablespoon honey

1 teaspoon cinnamon powder

1 tablespoon almonds, chopped

1 tablespoon walnuts, chopped

¼ cup pistachios, chopped

Directions:

- Heat a pan over medium heat, add the figs and the rest of the ingredients except the yogurt, stir and cook for 5 minutes.

- Divide the yogurt into bowls, divide the figs, mix on top, toss gently, and serve.

Nutrition: calories 198, fat 4.2, fiber 6.3, carbs 42.1, protein 3.4

Mango and Spinach Bowls

Preparation Time: 5 minutes

Cooking Time: 0 minutes

Servings: 4

Ingredients:

1 cup baby arugula

1 cup baby spinach, chopped

1 mango, peeled and cubed

1 cup strawberries, halved

1 tablespoon hemp seeds

1 cucumber, sliced

1 tablespoon lime juice

1 tablespoon tahini paste

1 tablespoon water

Directions:

- In a salad bowl, mix the arugula with the rest of the ingredients except the tahini and water and toss.
- In a small bowl, combine the tahini with the water, whisk well, add to the salad, toss, divide into small bowls and serve for breakfast.

Nutrition: calories 211, fat 4.5, fiber 6.5, carbs 10.2, protein 3.5

Oregano Quinoa and Spinach Muffins

Preparation Time: 10 minutes

Cooking Time: 35 minutes

Servings: 6

Ingredients:

1 cup quinoa

2 cups water

1 cup spinach, torn

2 spring onions, chopped

2 eggs, whisked

¼ cup parmesan cheese, grated

½ teaspoon garlic powder

sea salt and black pepper to taste

2 teaspoons oregano, dried

cooking spray

Directions:

- Put the water in a pan, heat over medium heat, add the quinoa, bring to a simmer, cook for 10 minutes, take off the heat, fluff with a fork and transfer to a bowl.

- Add the rest of the ingredients except the cooking spray and stir well.

- Grease a muffin tin with the cooking spray, divide the quinoa and spinach mix, Place into the oven at 350 degrees F and bake for 25 minutes.

- Serve the muffins warm for breakfast.

Nutrition: calories 267, fat 11.2, fiber 2.3, carbs 8.5, protein 4.5

Apricots Couscous

Preparation Time: 15 minutes

Cooking Time: 4 minutes

Servings: 4

Ingredients:

3 cups almond milk

1 teaspoon cinnamon powder

1 cup apricots, chopped

1 cup couscous, uncooked

3 teaspoons honey

4 teaspoons avocado oil

Directions:

- Heat a pan with the milk over medium heat, add the cinnamon and the rest of the ingredients, toss, and simmer for 4 minutes.
- Divide the mix into bowls, set aside for 15 minutes and serve for breakfast.

Nutrition: calories 617, fat 44, fiber 7.1, carbs 52.3, protein 10.2

Tapioca Pudding

Preparation Time: 30 minutes

Cooking Time: 15 minutes

Servings: 3

Ingredients:

¼ cup pearl tapioca

¼ cup maple syrup

2 cups almond milk

½ cup coconut flesh, shredded

1 and ½ teaspoon lemon juice

Directions:

- In a pan, combine the milk with the tapioca and the rest of the ingredients, bring to a simmer over medium heat, and cook for 15 minutes.
- Divide the mix into bowls, cool it down and serve for breakfast.

Nutrition: calories 361, fat 28.5, fiber 2.7, carbs 28.3, protein 2.8

Banana and Quinoa Casserole

Preparation Time: 10 minutes

Cooking Time: 1 hour and 20 minutes

Servings: 8

Ingredients:

3 cups bananas, peeled and mashed

¼ cup pure maple syrup

¼ cup molasses

1 tablespoon cinnamon powder

2 teaspoons vanilla extract

1 teaspoon cloves, ground

1 teaspoon ginger, ground

½ teaspoon allspice, ground

1 cup quinoa

¼ cup almonds, chopped

2 and ½ cups almond milk

Directions:

- In a baking dish, combine the bananas with the maple syrup, molasses, and the rest of the ingredients, toss and bake at 350 degrees F for 1 hour and 20 minutes.
- Divide the mix between plates and serve for breakfast.

Nutrition: calories 213, fat 4.1, fiber 4, carbs 41, protein 4.5

Spiced Chickpeas Bowls

Preparation Time: 10 minutes

Cooking Time: 30 minutes

Servings: 4

Ingredients:

15 ounces canned chickpeas, drained and rinsed

¼ teaspoon cardamom, ground

½ teaspoon cinnamon powder

1 and ½ teaspoons turmeric powder

1 teaspoon coriander, ground

1 tablespoon olive oil

pinch of salt and black pepper

¾ cup Greek yogurt

½ cup green olives pitted and halved

½ cup cherry tomatoes halved

1 cucumber, sliced

Directions:

- Spread the chickpeas on a lined baking sheet, add the cardamom, cinnamon, turmeric, coriander, oil, salt, and pepper, toss and bake at 375 degrees F for 30 minutes.
- In a bowl, combine the roasted chickpeas with the rest of the ingredients, toss and serve for breakfast.

Nutrition: calories 519, fat 34.5, fiber 13.3, carbs 49.8, protein 12

Avocado Spread

Preparation Time: 5 minutes

Cooking Time: 0 minutes

Servings: 8

Ingredients:

2 avocados, peeled, pitted and roughly chopped

1 tablespoon sun-dried tomatoes, chopped

2 tablespoons lemon juice

3 tablespoons cherry tomatoes, chopped

¼ cup red onion, chopped

1 teaspoon oregano, dried

2 tablespoons parsley, chopped

4 kalamata olives, pitted and chopped

pinch of salt and black pepper

Directions:

- Put the avocados in a bowl and mash with a fork.
- Add the rest of the ingredients, stir to combine and serve as a morning spread.

Nutrition: calories 110, fat 10, fiber 3.8, carbs 5.7, protein 1.2

Greek Beans Tortillas

Preparation Time: 5 minutes

Cooking Time: 20 minutes

Servings: 4

Ingredients:

1 red onion, chopped

2 garlic cloves, minced

1 tablespoon olive oil

1 green bell pepper, sliced

3 cups canned pinto beans, drained and rinsed

2 red chili peppers, chopped

4 tablespoon parsley, chopped

1 teaspoon cumin, ground

pinch of salt and black pepper

4 whole wheat Greek tortillas

1 cup cheddar cheese, shredded

Directions:

- Heat a pan with the oil over medium heat, add the onion and sauté for 5 minutes.

- Add the rest of the ingredients except the tortillas and the cheese, stir and cook for 15 minutes.

- Divide these beans mix on each Greek tortilla; also divide the cheese, roll the tortillas, and serve for breakfast.

Nutrition: calories 673, fat 14.9, fiber 23.7, carbs 75.4, protein 39

Ham & Egg Cups

Preparation Time: 15 minutes

Cooking Time: 30 minutes

Servings: 8

Ingredients:

cooked ham - deli-style (8 thin slices)

mozzarella cheese (.25 cups/1 oz.)

eggs (8)

optional: basil (8 tsp.)

black pepper (to taste)

grape or cherry tomatoes (6/as desired)

Also needed: muffin tin (8-count)

Directions:

- Program oven setting to 350° Fahrenheit. Coat the muffin tin cups with spray.

- Press the ham slice into the bottom and add the cheese to each prepared cups. Break an egg into the cup and sprinkle with pepper. Add the pesto if using it. Slice the tomatoes into halves and place them on each cup.

- Bake them for 18 to 20 minutes. The egg whites should be set, similar to a regular poached egg. Leave them in the cups for three to five minutes.

- Carefully take the cups out of the tin and serve.

Nutrition: Calories: 145 Protein: 11 grams Fat: 10 grams

Spinach and Artichoke Frittata

Preparation Time: 15 minutes

Cooking Time: 20 minutes

Servings: 4-6

Ingredients

10 large free-range eggs

1/2 cup sour cream

1 tablespoon Dijon mustard

1 teaspoon salt

1/4 teaspoon freshly ground black pepper

1 cup grated Parmesan cheese, divided

2 tablespoons olive oil

14 oz. marinated artichoke hearts, drained, patted dry, and quartered

5 oz. baby spinach

2 cloves garlic, minced

Directions:

- Preheat your oven to 400°F.
- Take a large bowl and add the eggs, sour cream, mustard, salt, pepper and ½ of the parmesan. Whisk to combine.
- Pop a skillet over a medium heat and add the oil.
- Add the artichokes and cook for 5 minutes until soft.
- Add the spinach and garlic, toss and cook for a further 2 minutes.
- Spread over the skillet then pour in the egg until the veggies

are covered.

- Top with the remaining Parmesan then cook for 2-3 minutes until the edges start to set.

- Pop into the oven and cook for 12-15 minutes until cooked to perfection.

- Remove from oven, let cool for 5 minutes, then serve and enjoy.

Nutrition: Calories: 185 Net carbs: 7g Fat: 13g Protein: 11

Avocado and Egg Breakfast Pizza

Preparation Time: 15 minutes

Cooking Time: 20 minutes

Servings: 4

Ingredients

1 large Hass avocado

1 tablespoon finely chopped cilantro

1 1/2 teaspoons lime juice

1/8 teaspoon salt

1/2 lb. pizza dough, homemade or store-bought

4 large eggs

1 tablespoon vegetable oil

hot sauce (optional)

Directions:

- Take a medium bowl and add the avocado, cilantro, lime juice and salt. Mash well until smooth.

- Take the pizza dough and divide into 4 equal pieces.

- Using a dusting of flour and a rolling pin, roll out into a circle approx. 6" wide.

- Take a skillet then lightly oil.

- Place the dough in the skillet and cook for a few minutes on each side until fluffy.

- Repeat with the remaining dough.

- Divide the avocado mixture between the pizzas and spread to cover.

- Add more oil to the pan then cook the eggs until exactly as you like them.

- Remove from the pan and place on the pizzas.

- Serve and enjoy.

Nutrition: Calories: 400 Net carbs: 50g Fat: 23g Protein: 3g

Spinach Feta Breakfast Wraps

Preparation Time: 15 minutes

Cooking Time: 20 minutes

Servings: 4

Ingredients

10 large free-range eggs

1/2 lb. baby spinach

4 large whole-wheat tortillas

1/2-pint cherry or grape tomatoes, halved

4 oz. feta cheese, crumbled

butter or olive oil, to taste

salt and pepper, to taste

Directions:

- Take a large bowl and add the eggs. Whisk well.

- Pop a skillet over a medium heat and add enough butter or oil to cover the bottom of the pan.

- Add the eggs and cook to perfection.

- Remove from the pan and leave to cool slightly.

- Add a touch more oil or butter to the pan then add the spinach, cooking until wilted.

- Pop your tortilla wraps into the microwave for a few seconds until warm.

- Place the wrap onto a flat surface then top with eggs, spinach, tomato and feta.

- Wrap then repeat with the remaining tortillas.

- Serve and enjoy.

Nutrition: Calories: 1061 Net carbs: 77g Fat: 68g Protein: 55g

Summer Vegetables with Eggs

Preparation Time: 5 minutes

Cooking Time: 30 minutes

Servings: 2

Ingredients

1 tablespoon olive oil

1 small yellow onion, halved and thinly sliced

1 clove garlic, minced

2 medium summer squash or zucchini

2 medium tomatoes, chopped

1/2 teaspoon fresh thyme

1 teaspoon ground Spanish piquillo pepper or Spanish paprika

1 medium red bell pepper

salt and pepper, to taste

2 large free-range eggs

Directions:

- Place a skillet over medium heat, then add the olive oil.

- Add the onion and cook for five minutes until soft.

- Throw in the garlic and cook for a further minute.

- Add the squash or zucchini and cook for 10 minutes until it begins to get soft.

- Add the tomatoes, thyme, and paprika and leave to cook for 20 minutes until thick.

- Meanwhile, roast your pepper by popping it onto a fork and holding it over a naked flame for a minute or two until the skin begins to blacken and burn.

- Leave to cool slightly, then remove the core and seeds and chop into 1" chunks.

- Take the skillet from the heat and add the roasted peppers and salt and pepper. Let cool.

- Place another skillet over medium heat, add the oil, then cook your eggs exactly as you like them.

- Serve everything together and enjoy.

Nutrition: Calories: 212 Net carbs: 17g Fat: 13g Protein: 10g

Crispy White Beans with Greens and Poached Egg

Preparation Time: 15 minutes

Cooking Time: 20 minutes

Servings: 4

Ingredients

3 tablespoons olive oil, divided

1 x 15 oz. can cannellini beans, drained and rinsed

1 teaspoon kosher salt, divided

2 teaspoons za'atar, divided

10 oz. Swiss chard stems removed and leaves thinly sliced

2 cloves garlic, minced

1/4 teaspoon red pepper flakes, plus more for Servings

1 tablespoon freshly squeezed lemon juice

4 large eggs, poached

Directions:

- Place a large skillet over medium heat and add 2 tablespoons of oil.
- Throw in the beans and cook for 2-4 minutes until starting to brown.
- Add ½ teaspoon of salt and 1 teaspoon of the za'atar and stir well.
- Continue to cook the beans for 3-5 minutes more until blistering.
- Add the remaining oil, throw in the chard, remaining salt, remaining za'atar garlic, and red pepper flakes. Stir well and cook for five minutes.
- Remove from heat, add the lemon juice and stir well.
- Serve topped with a poached egg and more red pepper flakes.
- Enjoy!

Nutrition: Calories: 187 Net carbs: 6g Fat: 15g Protein: 8g

Caprese Avocado Toast

Preparation Time: 5 minutes

Cooking Time: 10 minutes

Servings: 2

Ingredients

2 slices hearty sandwich bread

1 medium avocado, halved and pit removed

8 grape tomatoes, halved

12 bite-sized mozzarella balls

4 large fresh basil leaves, torn

2 tablespoons balsamic glaze

Directions:

- Toast the bread however you like.

- Meanwhile, mash the avocado well.

- When the toast is ready, spread the avocado over the top.

- Add tomatoes, mozzarella and basil, drizzle with the balsamic glaze, then serve and enjoy.

Nutrition: Calories: 187 Net carbs: 6g Fat: 15g Protein: 8g

'Huevos' Rancheros

Preparation Time: 10 minutes

Cooking Time: 15 minutes

Servings: 6

Ingredients:

salsa - ex. Old El Paso (16 oz. jar)

eggs (6)

flour tortillas/soft tacos (6-inch)

shredded cheese (.75 cup)

Also needed: 10-inch skillet

Directions:

- Heat the salsa until bubbly. Gently crack the eggs into the skillet.

- Place a top on the pot and simmer at med-low temperature for six to seven minutes. The eggs should be thoroughly cooked.

- Warm the tortillas and serve using a sprinkle of cheese.
- Spoon one egg onto each of the salsa-filled tortillas and serve.

Nutrition: Calories: 240 Protein: 11 grams Fat: 12 grams

Marinara Eggs with Parsley - Gluten-free

Preparation Time: 10 minutes

Cooking Time: 20 minutes

Servings: 6

Ingredients:

olive oil (1 tbsp.)

eggs (6 large)

medium onion (half of 1 or 1 cup)

garlic (2 cloves or 1 tsp.)

diced tomatoes - undrained - no-salt-added (2 - 14.5 oz. cans)

chopped Italian fresh flat-leaf parsley (.5 cup)

optional: crusty Italian bread with grated Parmesan or Romano cheese

Directions:

- Heat a skillet at a med-high temperature. Add the oil.

- Dice and toss the onions into the skillet. Sauté them for about five minutes. Stir occasionally and fold in the minced garlic, continuing to stir for another minute.

- Pour in the tomatoes with juices into the pan and let simmer until bubbling or for two to three minutes. Crack an egg into a coffee mug.

- Once the tomatoes are boiling, lower the heat to medium. Use the spoon to make six indentions in the tomato mixture.

- Add the egg to one of the slots and continue until you've used all the eggs.

- Place a lid on the pot and cook for six to seven minutes or until done.

- Garnish with the parsley and serve with bread and grated cheese to your liking.

Nutrition: Calories: 122 Protein: 7 grams Fat: 7 grams

Nutty Orange Polenta

Preparation Time: 10 minutes

Cooking Time: 15 minutes

Servings: 6

Ingredients:

plain polenta (2- 18-oz. tubes)

2% milk - divided (2.25 - 2.5 cups)

oranges (2)

pecans (.5 cup)

2% plain Greek yogurt (.25 cup)

honey (8 tsp.)

Directions:

- Slice the polenta into rounds and place in a microwavable dish to heat for 45 seconds.

- Prepare a pot using the medium heat setting and add the polenta. Mash it until roughly mashed.

- In a microwavable dish, pour in the milk and heat for one minute.

- Pour two cups of warm milk into the pot with the polenta and whisk thoroughly.

- Add in milk a few tablespoons at a time until it's the way you like it. Let the mixture cook slowly for about five minutes. Take the pan off the burner.

- Peel and chop the onions and pecans.

- Serve garnished with the oranges, pecans, honey, and yogurt.

Nutrition: Calories: 234 Protein: 3 grams Fat: 7 grams

Feta & Quinoa Egg Muffins

Preparation Time: 20 minutes

Cooking Time: 45-50 minutes

Servings: 12

Ingredients:

cooked quinoa (1 cup)

chopped baby spinach (2 cups)

Kalamata olives (.5 cup)

tomatoes (1 cup)

white onion (.5 cup)

fresh oregano (1 tbsp.)

salt (.5 tsp.)

olive oil (2 tsp.+ more for coating pans)

eggs (8)

crumbled feta cheese (1 cup)

Also needed: 12-cup muffin tin

Directions:

- Heat the oven to 350° Fahrenheit.

- Lightly grease the muffin tray cups with a spritz of cooking oil.

- Prepare a skillet using the medium temperature setting and add the oil. When hot, toss in the onions and sauté for two minutes.

- Dump the tomatoes into the skillet and sauté for one minute.

Fold in the spinach and continue cooking until the leaves have wilted (1 min.).

- Transfer the pot to the countertop and add the oregano and olives. Set aside.

- Crack the eggs into a mixing bowl and use an immersion stick blender to mix them thoroughly. Add the cooked veggies in with the rest of the ingredients.

- Stir until combined and scoop the mixture into the greased muffin cups.

- Set the timer to bake the muffins for 30 minutes until the muffins are set and brown.

- Cool for about ten minutes.

Nutrition: Calories: 113 Protein: 7 grams Fat: 7 grams

5-Minute Heirloom Tomato & Cucumber Toast

Preparation Time: 10 minutes

Cooking Time: 6-10 minutes

Servings: 1

Ingredients:

Heirloom tomato (1 small)

Persian cucumber (1)

olive oil (1 tsp.)

oregano (1 pinch)

kosher salt and pepper (as desired)

low-fat whipped cream cheese (2 tsp.)

Trader Joe's Whole Grain Crispbread or your choice (2 pieces)

balsamic glaze (1 tsp.)

Directions:

- Dice the cucumber and tomato. Combine all of the fixings

except for the cream cheese.

- Smear the cheese on the bread and add the mixture (step 1).

- Top it off with the balsamic glaze and serve.

Nutrition: Protein: 3 grams Fat: 8 grams Calories: 177

Garbanzo Bean Salad

Preparation Time: 10 minutes

Cooking Time: 0 minutes

Servings: 4

Ingredients:

1 and ½ cups cucumber, cubed

15 ounces canned garbanzo beans, drained and rinsed

3 ounces black olives, pitted and sliced

1 tomato, chopped

¼ cup red onion, chopped

5 cups salad greens

pinch of salt and black pepper

½ cup feta cheese, crumbled

3 tablespoons olive oil

1 tablespoon lemon juice

¼ cup parsley, chopped

Directions:

- In a salad bowl, combine garbanzo beans with the cucumber, tomato, and the rest of the ingredients except the cheese; toss.

- Divide the mix into small bowls, sprinkle the cheese on top and serve for breakfast.

Nutrition: calories 268, fat 16, fiber 7, carbs 24, protein 9

Brown Rice Salad

Preparation Time: 10 minutes

Cooking Time: 0 minutes

Servings: 4

Ingredients:

9 ounces brown rice, cooked

7 cups baby arugula

15 ounces canned garbanzo beans, drained and rinsed

4 ounces feta cheese, crumbled

¾ cup basil, chopped

pinch of salt and black pepper

2 tablespoons lemon juice

¼ teaspoon lemon zest, grated

¼ cup olive oil

Directions:

- In a salad bowl, combine the brown rice with the arugula, the beans and the rest of the ingredients.
- Toss and serve cold for breakfast.

Nutrition: calories 473, fat 22, fiber 7, carbs 53, protein 13

Tahini Pine Nuts Toast

Preparation Time: 5 minutes

Cooking Time: 0 minutes

Servings: 2

Ingredients:

2 whole wheat bread slices, toasted

1 teaspoon water

1 tablespoon tahini paste

2 teaspoons feta cheese, crumbled

juice of ½ lemon

2 teaspoons pine nuts

pinch of black pepper

Directions:

- In a bowl, mix the tahini with the water and the lemon juice, whisk well and spread over the toasted bread slices.

- Top each servings with remaining ingredients and serve for breakfast.

Nutrition: calories 142, fat 7.6, fiber 2.7, carbs 13.7, protein 5.8

Feta - Avocado & Mashed Chickpea Toast

Preparation Time: 10 minutes

Cooking Time: 15 minutes

Servings: 4

Ingredients:

chickpeas (15 oz. can)

diced feta cheese (2 oz. - .5 cup)

pitted avocado (1)

fresh juice: lemon (2 tsp.) or orange (1 tbsp.)

black pepper (.5 tsp.)

honey (2 tsp.)

multigrain toast (4 slices)

Directions:

- Toast the bread. Drain the chickpeas in a colander. Scoop the avocado flesh into the bowl.

- Use a large fork/potato masher to mash them until mix is

spreadable.

- Pour in the lemon juice, pepper, and the feta.

- Combine and divide onto the four slices of toast.

- Drizzle with honey and serve.

Nutrition: Calories: 337 Protein: 13 grams Fat: 13 grams

Stuffed Pita Breads

Preparation Time: 5 minutes

Cooking Time: 15 minutes

Servings: 4

Ingredients:

1 and ½ tablespoons olive oil

1 tomato, cubed

1 garlic clove, minced

1 red onion, chopped

¼ cup parsley, chopped

15 ounces canned fava beans, drained and rinsed

¼ cup lemon juice

salt and black pepper to taste

4 whole wheat pita bread pockets

Directions:

- Heat a pan with the oil over medium heat, add the onion, stir and sauté for 5 minutes.

- Add the rest of the ingredients, stir and cook for 10 minutes more

- Stuff the pita pockets with mix and serve for breakfast.

Nutrition: calories 382, fat 1.8, fiber 27.6, carbs 66, protein 28.5

Blueberries Quinoa

Preparation Time: 5 minutes

Cooking Time: 0 minutes

Servings: 4

Ingredients:

2 cups almond milk

2 cups quinoa, already cooked

½ teaspoon cinnamon powder

1 tablespoon honey

1 cup blueberries

¼ cup walnuts, chopped

Directions:

- In a bowl, mix the quinoa with the milk and the rest of the ingredients, toss, divide into smaller bowls and serve for breakfast.

Nutrition: calories 284, fat 14.3, fiber 3.2, carbs 15.4, protein 4.4

Endives, Fennel and Orange Salad

Preparation Time: 5 minutes

Cooking Time: 0 minutes

Servings: 4

Ingredients:

1 tablespoon balsamic vinegar

2 garlic cloves, minced

1 teaspoon Dijon mustard

2 tablespoons olive oil

1 tablespoon lemon juice

sea salt and black pepper to taste

½ cup black olives, pitted and chopped

1 tablespoon parsley, chopped

7 cups baby spinach

2 endives, shredded

3 medium navel oranges, peeled and cut into segments

2 bulbs fennel, shredded

Directions:

- In a salad bowl, combine the spinach with the endives, oranges, fennel and the rest of the ingredients.

- Toss and serve for breakfast.

Nutrition: calories 97, fat 9.1, fiber 1.8, carbs 3.7, protein 1.9

Raspberries and Yogurt Smoothie

Preparation Time: 5 minutes

Cooking Time: 0 minutes

Servings: 2

Ingredients:

2 cups raspberries

½ cup Greek yogurt

½ cup almond milk

½ teaspoon vanilla extract

Directions:

- In a blender, combine the raspberries with the milk, vanilla and the yogurt, pulse well.

- Divide into 2 glasses and serve for breakfast.

Nutrition: calories 245, fat 9.5, fiber 2.3, carbs 5.6, protein 1.6

Homemade Muesli

Preparation Time: 15 minutes

Cooking Time: 20 minutes

Servings: 8

Ingredients

3 1/2 cups rolled oats

1/2 cup wheat bran

1/2 teaspoon kosher salt

1/2 teaspoon ground cinnamon

1/2 cup sliced almonds

1/4 cup raw pecans, coarsely chopped

1/4 cup raw pepitas (shelled pumpkin seeds)

1/2 cup unsweetened coconut flakes

1/4 cup dried apricots, coarsely chopped

1/4 cup dried cherries

Directions:

- Take a medium bowl and combine the oats, wheat bran, salt and cinnamon. Stir well.
- Place the mixture onto a baking sheet.
- Next place the almonds, pecans and pepitas onto another baking sheet and toss.
- Pop both trays into the oven and heat to 350°F.
- Bake for 10-12 minutes.
- Remove from the oven and set to one side.
- Let the nuts to cool but take the one with the oats, sprinkle with the coconut and pop back into the oven for 5 minutes more.
- Remove and let to cool.

- In a large bowl, combine the contents of both trays then stir well to combine.

- Throw in the apricots and cherries and stir well.

- Pop into an airtight container until to be used.

Nutrition: Calories: 250 Net carbs: 36g Fat: 10g Protein: 7g

Tangerine and Pomegranate Breakfast Fruit Salad

Preparation Time: 15 minutes

Cooking Time: 20 minutes

Servings: 5

Ingredients

For the grains:

1 cup pearl or hulled barley

3 cups water

3 tablespoons olive oil, divided

1/2 teaspoon kosher salt

For the fruit...

1/2 large pineapple, peeled and cut into 1 ½" chunks

6 tangerines

1 1/4 cups pomegranate seeds

1 small bunch fresh mint

For the dressing:

1/3 cup honey

juice and finely grated zest of 1 lemon

juice and finely grated zest of 2 limes

1/2 teaspoon kosher salt

1/4 cup olive oil

1/4 cup toasted hazelnut oil (olive oil is fine too)

Directions:

- Place the grain into a strainer and rinse well.
- Take 2 baking sheets, line with paper, and add the grain. Spread well to cover, then let dry.
- Next, place the water into a saucepan and place over medium heat.
- Place a skillet over medium heat, add 2 tablespoons of the oil, add the barley, and toas for 2 minutes.
- Add the water and salt and bring to a boil.
- Reduce to simmer and cook for 40 minutes until most of the liquid has been absorbed.
- Turn off the heat and let stand for 10 minutes to steam cook the rest.
- Meanwhile, take a medium bowl and add the honey, juices, zest, and salt, and stir well.
- Add the olive oil, then nut oil and stir again. Pop into the fridge until needed.
- Remove the lid from the barley, then place on another prepared baking sheet and let cool.
- Drizzle with oil and let cool completely, then pop into the fridge.
- When ready to serve, divide the grains, pineapple, orange, pomegranate, and mint between the bowls.
- Drizzle with the dressing, then serve and enjoy.

Nutrition: Calories: 400 Net carbs: 50g Fat: 23g Protein: 3g

Chapter 2:
Side Dishes

Bulgur, Kale and Cheese Mix

Preparation Time: 10 minutes

Cooking Time: 10 minutes

Servings: 6

Ingredients:

4 ounces bulgur wheat

4 ounces kale, chopped

1 tablespoon mint, chopped

3 spring onions, chopped

1 cucumber, chopped

pinch of allspice, ground

2 tablespoons olive oil

zest and juice of ½ lemon

4 ounces feta cheese, crumbled

Directions:

- Put bulgur in a bowl, cover with hot water, set aside for 10 minutes and fluff with a fork.

- Heat a pan with the oil over medium heat, add the onions and allspice and cook for 3 minutes.

- Add the bulgur and the rest of the ingredients, cook everything for 5-6 minutes more, divide between plates, and serve.

Nutrition: calories 200, fat 6.7, fiber 3.4, carbs 15.4, protein 4.5

Spicy Green Beans Mix

Preparation Time: 5 minutes

Cooking Time: 15 minutes

Servings: 4

Ingredients:

4 teaspoons olive oil

1 garlic clove, minced

½ teaspoon hot paprika

¾ cup veggie stock

1 yellow onion, sliced

1 pound green beans, trimmed and halved

½ cup goat cheese, shredded

2 teaspoon balsamic vinegar

Directions:

- Heat a pan with the oil over medium heat, add the garlic, stir and cook for 1 minute.
- Add the green beans and the rest of the ingredients, toss, cook everything for 15 minutes more.
- Divide between plates and serve as a side dish.

Nutrition: calories 188, fat 4, fiber 3, carbs 12.4, protein 4.4

Beans and Rice

Preparation Time: 10 minutes

Cooking Time: 55 minutes

Servings: 6

Ingredients:

1 tablespoon olive oil

1 yellow onion, chopped

2 celery stalks, chopped

2 garlic cloves, minced

2 cups brown rice

1 and ½ cup canned black beans, rinsed and drained

4 cups water

salt and black pepper to taste

Directions:

- Heat a pan with the oil over medium heat, add the celery, garlic and the onion, stir and cook for 10 minutes.

- Add the rest of the ingredients, stir, bring to a simmer and cook over medium heat for 45 minutes.

- Divide between plates and serve.

Nutrition: calories 224, fat 8.4, fiber 3.4, carbs 15.3, protein 6.2

Lime Cucumber Mix

Preparation Time: 10 minutes

Cooking Time: 0 minutes

Servings: 8

Ingredients:

4 cucumbers, chopped

½ cup green bell pepper, chopped

1 yellow onion, chopped

1 chili pepper, chopped

1 garlic clove, minced

1 teaspoon parsley, chopped

2 tablespoons lime juice

1 tablespoon dill, chopped

Salt and black pepper to taste

1 tablespoon olive oil

Directions:

- In a large bowl, mix the cucumber with the bell peppers and the rest of the ingredients.

- Toss and serve as a side dish.

Nutrition: calories 123, fat 4.3, fiber 2.3, carbs 5.6, protein 2

Walnuts Cucumber Mix

Preparation Time: 5 minutes

Cooking Time: 0 minutes

Servings: 2

Ingredients:

2 cucumbers, chopped

1 tablespoon olive oil

salt and black pepper to taste

1 red chili pepper, dried

1 tablespoon lemon juice

3 tablespoons walnuts, chopped

1 tablespoon balsamic vinegar

1 teaspoon chives, chopped

Directions:

- In a bowl, mix the cucumbers with the oil and the rest of the ingredients.

- Toss and serve as a side dish.

Nutrition: calories 121, fat 2.3, fiber 2.0, carbs 6.7, protein 2.4

Cheesy Beet Salad

Preparation Time: 10 minutes

Cooking Time: 1 hour

Servings: 4

Ingredients:

4 beets, peeled and cut into wedges

3 tablespoons olive oil

salt and black pepper to taste

¼ cup lime juice

8 slices goat cheese, crumbled

1/3 cup walnuts, chopped

1 tablespoons chives, chopped

Directions:

- In a roasting pan, combine the beets with the oil, salt and pepper, toss and bake at 400 degrees F for 1 hour.
- Cool the beets down, transfer them to a bowl, add the rest of the ingredients.
- Toss and serve as a side salad.

Nutrition: calories 156, fat 4.2, fiber 3.4, carbs 6.5, protein 4

Rosemary Beets

Preparation Time: 10 minutes

Cooking Time: 20 minutes

Servings: 4

Ingredients:

4 medium beets, peeled and cubed

1/3 cup balsamic vinegar

1 teaspoon rosemary, chopped

1 garlic clove, minced

½ teaspoon Italian seasoning

1 tablespoon olive oil

Directions:

- Heat a pan with the oil over medium heat, add the beets and the rest of the ingredients, toss, and cook for 20 minutes.

- Divide the mix between plates and serve as a side dish.

Nutrition: calories 165, fat 3.4, fiber 4.5, carbs 11.3, protein 2.3

Squash and Tomatoes Mix

Preparation Time: 10 minutes

Cooking Time: 20 minutes

Servings: 6

Ingredients:

5 medium squash, cubed

pinch of salt and black pepper

3 tablespoons olive oil

1 cup pine nuts, toasted

¼ cup goat cheese, crumbled

6 tomatoes, cubed

½ yellow onion, chopped

2 tablespoons cilantro, chopped

2 tablespoons lemon juice

Directions:

- Heat a pan with the oil over medium heat, add the onion and pine nuts and cook for 3 minutes.

- Add the squash and the rest of the ingredients, cook everything for 15 minutes, divide between plates and serve as a side dish.

Nutrition: calories 200, fat 4.5, fiber 3.4, carbs 6.7, protein 4

Balsamic Eggplant Mix

Preparation Time: 10 minutes

Cooking Time: 20 minutes

Servings: 6

Ingredients:

1/3 cup chicken stock

2 tablespoons balsamic vinegar

pinch of salt and black pepper

1 tablespoon lime juice

2 big eggplants, sliced

1 tablespoon rosemary, chopped

¼ cup cilantro, chopped

2 tablespoons olive oil

Directions:

- In a roasting pan, combine the eggplants with the stock, the vinegar and the rest of the ingredients.
- Place the pan in the oven and bake at 390 degrees F for 20 minutes.
- Divide the mixture between plates and serve as a side dish.

Nutrition: calories 201, fat 4.5, fiber 3, carbs 5.4, protein 3

Sage Barley Mix

Preparation Time: 10 minutes

Cooking Time: 45 minutes

Servings: 4

Ingredients:

1 tablespoon olive oil

1 red onion, chopped

1 tablespoon leaves, chopped

1 garlic clove, minced

14 ounces barley

½ tablespoon parmesan, grated

6 cups veggie stock

salt and black pepper to taste

Directions:

- Heat a pan with the oil over medium heat, add the onion and garlic, stir and sauté for 5 minutes.
- Add the sage, barley and the rest of the ingredients except the Parmesan, stir, bring to a simmer and cook for 40 minutes,
- Add the Parmesan, stir, divide between plates.

Nutrition: calories 210, fat 6.5, fiber 3.4, carbs 8.6, protein 3.4

Chickpeas and Beets Mix

Preparation Time: 10 minutes

Cooking Time: 25 minutes

Servings: 4

Ingredients:

3 tablespoons capers, drained and chopped

juice of 1 lemon

zest of 1 lemon, grated

1 red onion, chopped

3 tablespoons olive oil

14 ounces canned chickpeas, drained

8 ounces beets, peeled and cubed

1 tablespoon parsley, chopped

salt and pepper to taste

Directions:

- Heat a pan with the oil over medium heat, add the onion, lemon zest, lemon juice and the capers and sauté for 5 minutes.
- Add the rest of the ingredients, stir and cook over medium-low heat for 20 minutes more.
- Divide the mixture between plates and serve as a side dish.

Nutrition: calories 199, fat 4.5, fiber 2.3, carbs 6.5, protein 3.3

Creamy Sweet Potatoes Mix

Preparation Time: 10 minutes

Cooking Time: 1 hour

Servings: 4

Ingredients:

4 tablespoons olive oil

1 garlic clove, minced

4 medium sweet potatoes, pricked with a fork

1 red onion, sliced

3 ounces baby spinach

zest and juice of 1 lemon

small bunch dill, chopped

1 and ½ tablespoons Greek yogurt

2 tablespoons tahini paste

salt and black pepper to taste

Directions:

- Put the potatoes on a baking sheet lined with parchment paper, place in oven at 350 degrees F and cook for 1 hour.

- Peel the potatoes, cut into wedges and put them in a bowl.

- Add the garlic, the oil and the rest of the ingredients, toss, divide the mix between plates and serve.

Nutrition: calories 214, fat 5.6, fiber 3.4, carbs 6.5, protein 3.1

Cabbage and Mushrooms Mix

Preparation Time: 10 minutes

Cooking Time: 15 minutes

Servings: 2

Ingredients:

1 yellow onion, sliced

2 tablespoons olive oil

1 tablespoon balsamic vinegar

½ pound white mushrooms, sliced

1 green cabbage head, shredded

4 spring onions, chopped

salt and black pepper to taste

Directions:

- Heat a pan with the oil over medium heat, add the yellow onion and the spring onions and cook for 5 minutes.

- Add the rest of the ingredients, cook everything for 10 minutes, divide between plates and serve.

Nutrition: calories 199, fat 4.5, fiber 2.4, carbs 5.6, protein 2.2

Lemon Mushroom Rice

Preparation Time: 10 minutes

Cooking Time: 30 minutes

Servings: 4

Ingredients:

2 cups chicken stock

1 yellow onion, chopped

½ pound white mushrooms, sliced

2 garlic cloves, minced

8 ounces wild rice

juice and zest of 1 lemon

1 tablespoon chives, chopped

6 tablespoons goat cheese, crumbled

salt and black pepper to taste

Directions:

- Heat a pot with the stock over medium heat, add rice, onion and the rest of the ingredients except the chives and cheese, bring to a simmer and cook for 25 minutes.
- Add the remaining ingredients, cook everything for 5 minutes, divide between plates and serve as a side dish.

Nutrition: calories 222, fat 5.5, fiber 5.4, carbs 12.3, protein 5.6

Paprika and Chives Potatoes

Preparation Time: 10 minutes

Cooking Time: 1 hour and 8 minutes

Servings: 4

Ingredients:

4 potatoes, scrubbed and pricked with a fork

1 tablespoon olive oil

1 celery stalk, chopped

2 tomatoes, chopped

1 teaspoon sweet paprika

salt and black pepper to taste

2 tablespoons chives, chopped

Directions:

- Arrange the potatoes on a baking sheet lined with parchment paper, place in oven and bake at 350 degrees F for 1 hour.
- Cool potatoes down, peel and cut into larger cubes.
- Heat a pan with the oil over medium heat, add the celery and the tomatoes and sauté for 2 minutes.
- Add the potatoes and the rest of the ingredients, toss, cook everything for 6 minutes.
- Divide the mix between plates and serve as a side dish.

Nutrition: calories 233, fat 8.7, fiber 4.5, carbs 14.4, protein 6.4

Lemony Carrots

Preparation Time: 10 minutes

Cooking Time: 40 minutes

Servings: 4

Ingredients:

3 tablespoons olive oil

2 pounds baby carrots, trimmed

salt and black pepper to taste

½ teaspoon lemon zest, grated

1 tablespoon lemon juice

1/3 cup Greek yogurt

1 garlic clove, minced

1 teaspoon cumin, ground

1 tablespoon dill, chopped

Directions:

- In a roasting pan, combine the carrots with the oil, salt, pepper and the rest of the ingredients except the dill; toss and bake at 400 degrees F for 20 minutes.
- Reduce the temperature to 375 degrees F and cook for 20 minutes more.
- Divide the mix between plates, sprinkle the dill on top and serve.

Nutrition: calories 192, fat 5.4, fiber 3.4, carbs 7.3, protein 5.6

Tomato and Millet Mix

Preparation Time: 10 minutes

Cooking Time: 20 minutes

Servings: 6

Ingredients:

3 tablespoons olive oil

1 cup millet

2 spring onions, chopped

2 tomatoes, chopped

½ cup cilantro, chopped

1 teaspoon chili paste

6 cups cold water

½ cup lemon juice

salt and black pepper to taste

Directions:

- Heat a pan with the oil over medium heat, add the millet, stir and cook for 4 minutes.
- Add the water, salt and pepper, stir, bring to a simmer over medium heat cook for 15 minutes.

- Add the rest of the ingredients, toss, divide the mix between plates and serve as a side dish.

Nutrition: calories 222, fat 10.2, fiber 3.4, carbs 14.5, protein 2.4

Quinoa and Greens Salad

Preparation Time: 10 minutes

Cooking Time: 0 minutes

Servings: 4

Ingredients:

1 cup quinoa, cooked

1 medium bunch collard greens, chopped

4 tablespoons walnuts, chopped

2 tablespoons balsamic vinegar

4 tablespoons tahini paste

4 tablespoons cold water

pinch of salt and black pepper

1 tablespoon olive oil

Directions:

- In a bowl, mix the tahini with the water and vinegar and whisk.
- In a bowl, mix the quinoa with the rest of the ingredients and the tahini dressing.
- Toss, divide the mix between plates and serve as a side dish.

Nutrition: calories 175, fat 3, fiber 3, carbs 5, protein 3

Veggies and Avocado Dressing

Preparation Time: 10 minutes

Cooking Time: 0 minutes

Servings: 4

Ingredients:

3 tablespoons pepitas, roasted

3 cups water

2 tablespoons cilantro, chopped

4 tablespoons parsley, chopped

1 and ½ cups corn

1 cup radish, sliced

2 avocados, peeled, pitted and chopped

2 mangos, peeled and chopped

3 tablespoons olive oil

4 tablespoons Greek yogurt

1 teaspoons balsamic vinegar

2 tablespoons lime juice

salt and black pepper to taste

Directions:

- In a blender, mix the olive oil with avocados, salt, pepper, lime juice, the yogurt and the vinegar and pulse.

- In a bowl, mix the pepitas with the cilantro, parsley and the rest of the ingredients, and toss.

- Add the avocado dressing, toss, divide the mix between plates and serve as a side dish.

Nutrition: calories 403, fat 30.5, fiber 10, carbs 23.5, protein 3.5

Cauliflower Quinoa

Preparation Time: 5 minutes

Cooking Time: 10 minutes

Servings: 4

Ingredients:

1 and ½ cups quinoa, coked

3 tablespoons olive oil

3 cups cauliflower florets

2 spring onions, chopped

salt and pepper to taste

1 tablespoon red wine vinegar

1 tablespoon parsley, chopped

1 tablespoon chives, chopped

Directions:

- Heat a pan with the oil over medium-high heat, add the spring onions and cook for 2 minutes.
- Add the cauliflower, quinoa and the rest of the ingredients, toss, cook over medium heat for 8-9 minutes.
- Divide between plates and serve as a side dish.

Nutrition: calories 220, fat 16.7, fiber 5.6, carbs 6.8, protein 5.4

Mixed Veggies and Chard

Preparation Time: 10 minutes

Cooking Time: 20 minutes

Servings: 4

Ingredients:

½ cup celery, chopped

½ cup carrot, chopped

½ cup red onion, chopped

½ cup red bell pepper, chopped

1 tablespoon olive oil

1 cup veggie stock

½ cup black olives, pitted and chopped

10 ounces ruby chard, torn

salt and black pepper to taste

1 teaspoon balsamic vinegar

Directions:

- Heat a pan with the oil over medium-high heat, add the celery, carrot, onion, bell pepper, salt and pepper, stir and sauté for 5 minutes.

- Add the rest of the ingredients, toss, cook over medium heat for 15 minutes more.

- Divide between plates and serve as a side dish.

Nutrition: calories 150, fat 6.7, fiber 2.6, carbs 6.8, protein 5.4

Spicy Broccoli and Almonds

Preparation Time: 10 minutes

Cooking Time: 30 minutes

Servings: 4

Ingredients:

1 broccoli head, florets separated

2 garlic cloves, minced

1 tablespoon olive oil

1 tablespoon chili powder

salt and black pepper to taste

1 tablespoon mint, chopped

2 tablespoons almonds, toasted and chopped

Directions:

- In a roasting pan, combine the broccoli with the garlic, oil and the rest of the ingredients, toss, Place in the oven and cook at 390 degrees F for 30 minutes.

- Divide the mix between plates and serve as a side dish.

Nutrition: calories 156, fat 5.4, fiber 1.2, carbs 4.3, protein 2

Balsamic Asparagus

Preparation Time: 10 minutes

Cooking Time: 15 minutes

Servings: 4

Ingredients:

3 tablespoons olive oil

3 garlic cloves, minced

2 tablespoons shallot, chopped

salt and black pepper to taste

2 teaspoons balsamic vinegar

1 and ½ pound asparagus, trimmed

Directions:

- Heat a pan with the oil over medium-high heat, add the garlic and the shallot and sauté for 3 minutes.

- Add the rest of the ingredients, cook for 12 minutes more, divide between plates and serve as a side dish.

Nutrition: calories 100, fat 10.5, fiber 1.2, carbs 2.3, protein 2.1

Chapter 3:
Lunch

Avocado & Tuna Tapas

Preparation Time: 10 minutes

Cooking Time: 10 minutes

Servings: 4

Ingredients:

solid white tuna packed in water (12 oz. can)

green onions (3 + more for garnish)

red bell pepper (half of 1)

garlic salt and black pepper (as desired)

mayonnaise (1 tbsp.)

balsamic vinegar (1 dash)

ripe avocados (2)

Directions:

- Drain the tuna thoroughly. Remove the pit and slice the avocados into halves.

- Chop the bell pepper, and thinly slice the onions. Whisk the vinegar, red pepper, onions, salt, pepper, mayonnaise, and tuna.

- Load the avocado halves with the tuna.

- Top off with a portion of green onions and black pepper before serving.

Nutrition: Calories: 194 Protein: 23.9 grams Fat: 18.2 grams

Greek Baked Zucchini & Potatoes

Preparation Time: 30 minutes

Cooking Time: 2 hours

Servings: 4

Ingredients:

potatoes (2 lb.)

zucchini (4 large)

red onions (4 small)

ripe tomatoes (6 pureed)

olive oil (.5 cup)

optional: freshly chopped parsley (2 tbsp.)

black pepper & sea salt (to taste)

Also needed: 9 by 13-inch or larger baking dish

Directions:

- Thinly slice the zucchini, onions, and potatoes.
- Set the oven to 400° Fahrenheit.
- Chop and spread the red onions, zucchini, and potatoes in the baking pan.
- Cover with pureed tomatoes, parsley, and olive oil.
- Sprinkle using salt and pepper. Toss until evenly coated.
- Bake for approximately one hour or until veggies are moist and softened.
- Cool slightly and serve at room temperature.

Nutrition: Calories: 534 Protein: 11.3 grams Fat: 28.3 grams

Chickpeas Soup

Preparation Time: 10 minutes

Cooking Time: 1 hour

Servings: 4

Ingredients:

3 tomatoes, cubed

2 yellow onions, chopped

2 tablespoons olive oil

4 celery stalks, chopped

½ cup parsley, chopped

2 garlic cloves, minced

16 ounces canned chickpeas, drained and rinsed

6 cups water

1 teaspoon cumin, ground

juice of ½ lemon

1 teaspoon turmeric powder

½ teaspoon cinnamon powder

½ teaspoon ginger, grated

salt and black pepper to taste

Directions:

- Heat a pot with the oil over medium heat, add the onion and the garlic and sauté for 5 minutes.

- Add the tomatoes, celery, cumin, turmeric, cinnamon, and ginger, stir and sauté for 5 minutes more.

- Add the remaining ingredients, bring soup to a boil over medium heat and simmer for 50 minutes.

- Ladle the soup into bowls and serve.

Nutrition: calories 300, fat 15.4, fiber 4.5, carbs 29.5, protein 15.4

Tomato Soup

Preparation Time: 10 minutes

Cooking Time: 55 minutes

Servings: 8

Ingredients:

4 pounds tomatoes, halved

2 tablespoons olive oil

6 garlic cloves, minced

1 yellow onion, chopped

salt and black pepper to taste

4 cups chicken stock

½ teaspoon red pepper flakes

½ cup basil, chopped

½ cup parmesan, grated

Directions:

- Arrange tomatoes in a roasting pan, add half of the oil, salt, and pepper, toss, and bake at 400 degrees F for 20 minutes.
- Heat a pot with the rest of the oil over medium heat, add the onion and sauté for 5 minutes.
- Add the tomatoes and the rest of the ingredients except the basil and Parmesan, bring to a simmer, and cook for 30 minutes.
- Blend the soup using an immersion blender, add the basil and the Parmesan, stir, divide into bowls and serve.

Nutrition: calories 237, fat 10, fiber 3.4, carbs 15.3, protein 7.4

Oyster Stew

Preparation Time: 10 minutes

Cooking Time: 1 hour and 10 minutes

Servings: 6

Ingredients:

2 garlic cloves, minced

¼ cup jarred roasted red peppers

2 teaspoons oregano, chopped

1 pound lamb meat, ground

1 tablespoon red wine vinegar

salt and black pepper to taste

1 teaspoon red pepper flakes

2 tablespoons olive oil

1 and ½ cups chicken stock

36 oysters, shucked

1 and ½ cups canned black-eyed peas, drained

Directions:

- Heat a pot with the oil over medium heat, add the meat and the garlic and brown for 5 minutes.

- Add peppers and the rest of the ingredients, bring to a simmer for 15 minutes.

- Divide the stew into bowls and serve.

Nutrition: calories 264, fat 9.3, fiber 1.2, carbs 2.3, protein 1.2

Potatoes and Lentils Stew

Preparation Time: 10 minutes

Cooking Time: 35 minutes

Servings: 4

Ingredients:

4 cups water

1 cup carrots, sliced

1 yellow onion, chopped

1 tablespoon olive oil

1 cup celery, chopped

2 garlic cloves, minced

2 pounds gold potatoes, cubed

1 and ½ cup lentils, dried

½ teaspoon smoked paprika

½ teaspoon oregano, dried

salt and black pepper to taste

14 ounces canned tomatoes, chopped

½ cup cilantro, chopped

Directions:

- Heat a pot with the oil over medium-high heat, add the onion, garlic, celery, and carrots, stir and cook for 5 minutes.
- Add the rest of the ingredients except the cilantro, stir, bring to a simmer and cook over medium heat for 25 minutes.
- Add the cilantro, divide the stew into bowls and serve.

Nutrition: calories 325, fat 17.3, fiber 6.8, carbs 26.4, protein 16.4

Chicken Salad

Preparation Time: 30 minutes

Cooking Time: 45 minutes

Servings: 4

Ingredients:

1 and ½ pounds chicken breast, skinless, boneless

1 tablespoon dill, chopped

zest of 2 lemons, grated

Juice of 2 lemons

3 tablespoons olive oil

1 tablespoon oregano, chopped

3 tablespoons parsley, chopped

pinch of salt and black pepper

For the barley:

2 and ½ cups chicken stock

1 cup barley

1 teaspoon oregano, dried

zest of 1 lemon, grated

juice of 1 lemon

¼ cup olive oil

2 red leaf lettuce heads, chopped

1 red onion, sliced

1 pint cherry tomatoes, sliced

2 avocados, peeled, pitted and sliced

Directions:

- Put the chicken breasts in a bowl, add the dill, zest of 2 lemons, juice of 2 lemons, 3 tablespoons oil, 1 tablespoon oregano, parsley, salt and pepper. Toss, cover the bowl, and set aside for 30 minutes.

- Heat up grill over medium-high heat, add the chicken, cook for 6 minutes on each side, cool down, slice and put in a bowl.

- Put the stock in a pot, add the barley, salt and pepper, bring to a simmer over medium heat, cook for 45 minutes, drain and put in the same bowl with the chicken.

- Add the dried oregano, zest of 1 lemon, juice of 1 lemon, ¼ cup oil, the lettuce, onion, tomatoes and the avocados.

- Toss and serve.

Nutrition: calories 342, fat 17.4, fiber 16.5, carbs 27.7, protein 26.4

Chicken Skillet

Preparation Time: 10 minutes

Cooking Time: 35 minutes

Servings: 6

Ingredients:

6 chicken thighs, bone-in and skin-on

juice of 2 lemons

1 teaspoon oregano, dried

1 red onion, chopped

salt and black pepper to taste

1 teaspoon garlic powder

2 garlic cloves, minced

2 tablespoons olive oil

2 and ½ cups chicken stock

1 cup white rice

1 tablespoon oregano, chopped

1 cup green olives, pitted and sliced

1/3 cup parsley, chopped

½ cup feta cheese, crumbled

Directions:

- Heat a pan with the oil over medium heat, add the chicken thighs skin side down, cook for 4 minutes on each side and transfer to a plate.

- Add the garlic and the onion to the pan, stir and sauté for 5 minutes.

- Add the rice, salt, pepper, the stock, oregano, and lemon juice, stir, cook for 1-2 minutes more and take off heat.

- Add the chicken to the pan, place the pan in the oven and bake at 375 degrees F for 25 minutes.

- Add the cheese, olives and parsley, divide the whole mix between plates and serve for lunch.

Nutrition: calories 435, fat 18.5, fiber 13.6, carbs 27.8, protein 25.6

Green Beans & Feta

Preparation Time: 10 minutes

Cooking Time: 15 minutes

Servings: 8

Ingredients:

olive oil (2 tbsp.)

freshly trimmed green beans (1 lb.)

red onion (2 tbsp.)

tarragon vinegar (1 tbsp.)

salt (.5 tsp.)

pepper (.25 tsp.)

garlic (1 clove)

crumbled feta cheese (.5 cup or 2 oz.)

Also needed: 6-quart saucepan

Directions:

- Add one inch of water into the pan and add the beans.

- Finely chop the onion and garlic and add the rest of the fixings (omit the cheese); simmer for eight to ten minutes with lid off. Drain.

- Scoop the beans into a serving dish and add the cheese.

- Toss and serve warm.

Nutrition: Fat: 5 grams Protein: 2 grams Calories: 80

Kale - Mediterranean-Style

Preparation Time: 10 minutes

Cooking Time: 15 minutes

Servings: 6

Ingredients:

chopped kale (12 cups)

olive oil (1 tbsp./as needed)

minced garlic (1 tbsp.)

salt and black pepper (as preferred)

soy sauce (1 tsp.)

lemon juice (2 tbsp.)

Directions:

- Prepare a saucepan with a steamer insert. Pour in plenty of water to cover the bottom.

- Put a lid on the pot and boil using the high-temperature setting.

- Toss in the kale. Once it boils, set time for 7-10 minutes. Drain.

- Whisk the soy sauce, lemon juice, garlic, oil, black pepper, and salt. Toss in the steamed kale. Toss until coated and serve.

Nutrition: Calories: 91 Protein: 4.6 grams Fat: 3.2 grams

Mediterranean Endive Boats

Preparation Time: 10 minutes

Cooking Time: 10 minutes

Servings: 8

Ingredients:

chopped sun-dried tomatoes (.33 cup)

chickpeas (.66 cup)

olive oil (1 tbsp.)

crumbled feta (.25 cup)

chopped basil leaves (3)

balsamic reduction (2 tbsp.)

Directions:

- Rinse and drain the chickpeas.

- Combine the oil with the drained chickpeas and tomatoes.

- Cut the base of the endive and pull the leaves apart. (It should make eight.)

- Arrange the leaves on the serving platter and add the chickpea mixture.

- Garnish with the crumbled feta and top off with chopped basil and a spritz of balsamic reduction.

Nutrition: Calories: 715 Protein: 32 grams Fat: 30 grams

Salmon with Warm Tomato-Olive Salad

Preparation Time: 15 minutes

Cooking Time: 25 minutes

Servings: 4

Ingredients:

salmon fillets (4/approx. 4 oz./1.25-inches thick)

celery (1 cup)

medium tomatoes (2)

fresh mint (.25 cup)

Kalamata olives (.5 cup)

garlic (.5 tsp.)

salt (1 tsp. + more to taste)

honey (1 tbsp.)

red pepper flakes (.25 tsp.)

olive oil (2 tbsp. + more for the pan)

vinegar (1 tsp.)

Directions:

- Slice the tomatoes and celery into 1-inch pieces and mince the garlic. Chop the mint and the olives.

- Heat the oven at the broiler setting.

- Whisk the oil, vinegar, honey, red pepper flakes, and salt (1 tsp.). Brush the mixture onto the salmon.

- Line the broiler pan with a sheet of foil. Spritz the pan lightly with olive oil, and add the fillets (skin side downward).

- Broil for four to six minutes until well done.

- Meanwhile, make the tomato salad. Mix ½ teaspoon of the salt with the garlic.

- Prepare a small saucepan on the stovetop using med-high temperature. Pour in the rest of the oil and add the garlic mixture with the olives and one tablespoon of vinegar. Simmer for about three minutes.

- Prepare the serving dishes. Pour the bubbly mixture into the bowl and add the mint, tomato, and celery. Dust with the salt as desired and toss.

- When the salmon is done, serve with tomato salad.

Nutrition: Calories: 433 Protein: 38 grams Fat: 26 grams

Shrimp & Penne

Preparation Time: 20 minutes

Cooking Time: 35 minutes

Servings: 8

Ingredients:

penne pasta (16 oz. pkg.)

salt (.25 tsp.)

olive oil (2 tbsp.)

diced tomatoes (2 - 14.5 oz. cans)

garlic (1 tbsp.)

red onion (.25 cup)

white wine (.25 cup)

shrimp (1 lb.)

grated Parmesan cheese (1 cup)

Directions:

- Dice the red onion and garlic. Peel and devein the shrimp.

- Add salt to a large soup pot of water and seton stovetop to boil. Add the pasta and cook for nine to ten minutes. Drain thoroughly in a colander.

- Empty oil into a skillet. Warm it using the medium temperature setting.

- Toss in the garlic and onion and sauté until they're tender.

- Pour in the tomatoes and wine. Continue cooking for about ten minutes, stirring occasionally.

- Fold in the shrimp and continue cooking for about five minutes or until opaque.

- Combine the pasta and shrimp and top off with the cheese to serve.

Nutrition: Fat: 8.5 grams Protein: 24.5 grams Calories: 385

Tilapia with Avocado & Red Onion

Preparation Time: 5 minutes

Cooking Time: 15 minutes

Servings: 4

Ingredients:

olive oil (1 tbsp.)

sea salt (.25 tsp.)

fresh orange juice (1 tbsp.)

tilapia fillets (four 4 oz. - more rectangular than square)

red onion (.25 cup)

sliced avocado (1)

Also needed: 9-inch pie plate

Directions:

- Combine salt, juice, and oil to add into the pie dish. Work with one fillet at a time. Place it in the dish and coat all sides.

- Arrange the fillets in a wagon wheel formation. (Each of the fillets should be in the center of the dish with the other end draped over the edge.)

- Place a tablespoon of the onion on top of each fillet and fold the end into the center. Cover the dish with plastic wrap, leaving one corner open to vent the steam.

- Place in the microwave using the high heat setting for three minutes. It's done when the center can be easily flaked.

- Top the fillets off with avocado and serve.

Nutrition: Calories: 200 Protein: 22 grams Fat: 11 grams

Berries and Grilled Calamari

Preparation Time: 5 minutes

Cooking Time: 5 minutes

Servings: 4

Ingredients:

¼ cup dried cranberries

¼ cup extra virgin olive oil

¼ cup olive oil

¼ cup sliced almonds

½ lemon, juiced

¾ cup blueberries

1 ½ pounds calamari tube, cleaned

1 Granny Smith apple, sliced thinly

1 tablespoon fresh lemon juice

2 tablespoons apple cider vinegar

6 cups fresh spinach

Freshly grated pepper to taste

sea salt to taste

Directions for Cooking:

- In a small bowl, make the vinaigrette by mixing well the tablespoon of lemon juice, apple cider vinegar, and extra virgin olive oil. Season with pepper and salt to taste. Set aside.

- Turn on the grill to medium fire and let the grates heat up for a minute or two.

- In a large bowl, add olive oil and calamari tube. Season calamari generously with pepper and salt.

- Place seasoned and oiled calamari onto heated grate and grill until cooked or opaque. This is around two minutes per side.

- As you wait for the calamari to cook, combine almonds, cranberries, blueberries, spinach, and the thinly sliced apple in a large salad bowl. Toss to mix.

- Remove cooked calamari from grill and transfer on a chopping board. Cut into ¼-inch thick rings and throw into the salad bowl.

- Drizzle with vinaigrette and toss well to coat salad.

- Serve and enjoy!

Nutrition: Calories per Servings: 567 Fat: 24.5g Protein: 54.8g Carbs: 30.6g

---

Cajun Garlic Shrimp Noodle Bowl

Preparation Time: 7 minutes

Cooking Time: 15 minutes

Servings: 2

Ingredients:

½ teaspoon salt

1 onion, sliced

1 red pepper, sliced

1 tablespoon butter

1 teaspoon garlic granules

1 teaspoon onion powder

1 teaspoon paprika

2 large zucchinis, cut into noodle strips

20 jumbo shrimps, shells removed and deveined

3 cloves garlic, minced

3 tablespoon ghee

dash of cayenne pepper

dash of red pepper flakes

Directions for Cooking:

- Prepare the Cajun seasoning by mixing the onion powder, garlic granules, pepper flakes, cayenne pepper, paprika, and salt. Toss in the shrimp and coat with the seasoning.

- In a skillet, heat the ghee and sauté the garlic. Add in the red pepper and onions and continue sautéing for 4 minutes.

- Add the Cajun shrimp and cook until opaque. Set aside.

- In another pan, heat the butter and sauté the zucchini noodles for three minutes.

- Assemble by placing the Cajun shrimps on top of the zucchini noodles.

Nutrition: Calories per Servings: 712 Fat: 30.0g Protein: 97.8g Carbs: 20.2g

Tarragon Cod Fillets

Preparation Time: 10 minutes

Cooking Time: 12 minutes

Servings: 4

Ingredients:

4 cod fillets, boneless

¼ cup capers, drained

1 tablespoon tarragon, chopped

sea salt and black pepper to taste

2 tablespoons olive oil

2 tablespoons parsley, chopped

1 tablespoon olive oil

1 tablespoon lemon juice

Directions:

- Heat a pan with the oil over medium-high heat, add the fish and cook for 3 minutes on each side.

- Add the rest of the ingredients, cook everything for 7 minutes more, divide between plates and serve.

Nutrition: Calories 162 Fat 9.6 Fiber 4.3 Carbs 12.4 Protein 16.5

Salmon and Radish Mix

Preparation Time: 10 minutes

Cooking Time: 15 minutes

Servings: 4

Ingredients:

2 tablespoons olive oil

1 tablespoon balsamic vinegar

1 and ½ cup chicken stock

4 salmon fillets, boneless

2 garlic cloves, minced

1 tablespoon ginger, grated

1 cup radishes, grated

¼ cup scallions, chopped

Directions:

- Heat a pan with the oil over medium-high heat, add the salmon, cook for 4 minutes on each side and divide between plates.
- Add the vinegar and the rest of the ingredients to the pan, toss gently, cook for 10 minutes, add over the salmon and serve.

Nutrition: Calories 274 Fat 14.5 Fiber 3.5 Carbs 8.5 Protein 22.3

Smoked Salmon and Watercress Salad

Preparation Time: 5 minutes

Cooking Time: 0 minutes

Servings: 4

Ingredients:

2 bunches watercress

1 pound smoked salmon, skinless, boneless and flaked

2 teaspoons mustard

¼ cup lemon juice

½ cup Greek yogurt

salt and black pepper to taste

1 big cucumber, sliced

2 tablespoons chives, chopped

Directions:

- In a salad bowl, combine the salmon with the watercress and the rest of the ingredients.
- Toss and serve right away.

Nutrition: Calories 244 Fat 16.7 Fiber 4.5 Carbs 22.5 Protein 15.6

Salmon and Corn Salad

Preparation Time: 5 minutes

Cooking Time: 0 minutes

Servings: 4

Ingredients:

½ cup pecans, chopped

2 cups baby arugula

1 cup corn

¼ pound smoked salmon, skinless, boneless and cut into small chunks

2 tablespoons olive oil

2 tablespoon lemon juice

sea salt and black pepper to taste

Directions:

- In a salad bowl, combine the salmon with the corn and the rest of the ingredients.

- Toss, and serve right away.

Nutrition: Calories 284 Fat 18.4 Fiber 5.4 Carbs 22.6 Protein 17.4

Mediterranean Nachos

Preparation Time: 10 minutes

Cooking Time: 10 minutes

Servings: 6

Ingredients:

Kalamata olives (2 tbsp.)

sun-dried tomatoes in oil (2 tbsp. + 2 tsp. oil)

drained Roma small plum tomato (1 medium)

green onion (1 tbsp.)

tortilla chips (4 oz./30 chips approx.)

feta cheese (4 oz.)

Directions:

- Prep the fixings. Thinly slice/chop the onion olives and tomatoes. Mix the sun-dried tomatoes, olives, oil, onions, and plum tomato. Set aside for now.

- Place the tortillas (single-layered) on a microwavable platter. Crumble the feta over the chips.

- Cook in the microwave for one minute on high.

- Rotate the dish and continue cooking for another 30 to 60 seconds or until bubbly.

- Spoon the tomato mixture over the chops and serve.

Nutrition: Calories: 170 Protein: 4 grams Fat: 11 grams

Mediterranean Potatoes

Preparation Time: 15 minutes

Cooking Time: 45-50 minutes

Servings: 4

Ingredients:

medium potatoes (4-5)

olive oil (1 tbsp.)

butter (1 tbsp. - melted)

Greek seasoning (6 tsp.)

garlic seasoning (.125 tsp.)

Also needed: 9 x 13-inch casserole dish

Directions:

- Set the oven temperature to 350° Fahrenheit.
- Cube the potatoes and toss into the dish with the rest of the fixings.
- Bake for 30-40 minutes. Turn occasionally.
- Serve when the potatoes are browned to your liking.

Nutrition: Calories: 207.8 Protein: 3.8 grams Fat: 6.3 grams

Turkey Fritters and Sauce

Preparation Time: 10 minutes

Cooking Time: 30 minutes

Servings: 4

Ingredients:

2 garlic cloves, minced

1 egg

1 red onion, chopped

1 tablespoon olive oil

¼ teaspoon red pepper flakes

1 pound turkey meat, ground

½ teaspoon oregano, dried

cooking spray

For the sauce:

1 cup Greek yogurt

1 cucumber, chopped

1 tablespoon olive oil

¼ teaspoon garlic powder

2 tablespoons lemon juice

¼ cup parsley, chopped

Directions:

- Heat a pan with 1 tablespoon oil over medium heat, add the onion and the garlic, sauté for 5 minutes, cool down and transfer to a bowl.

- Add the meat, turkey, oregano, and pepper flakes, stir and shape medium fritters out of this mix.

- Heat up another pan greased with cooking spray over medium-high heat, add the turkey fritters and brown for 5 minutes on each side.

- Place the pan in oven and bake fritters at 375 degrees F for 15 minutes more.

- Meanwhile, in a bowl, mix the yogurt with the cucumber, oil, garlic powder, lemon juice and parsley and whisk really well.

- Divide the fritters between plates, spread the sauce all over, and serve for lunch.

Nutrition: calories 364, fat 16.8, fiber 5.5, carbs 26.8, protein 23.4

Stuffed Eggplants

Preparation Time: 10 minutes

Cooking Time: 35 minutes

Servings: 4

Ingredients:

2 eggplants, halved lengthwise and 2/3 of the flesh scooped out

3 tablespoons olive oil

1 red onion, chopped

2 garlic cloves, minced

1 pint white mushrooms, sliced

2 cups kale, torn

2 cups quinoa, cooked

1 tablespoon thyme, chopped

zest and juice of 1 lemon

salt and black pepper to taste

½ cup Greek yogurt

3 tablespoons parsley, chopped

Directions:

- Rub the inside of each eggplant half with half of the oil and arrange them on a baking sheet lined with parchment paper.

- Heat a pan with the rest of the oil over medium heat, add the onion and the garlic and sauté for 5 minutes.

- Add the mushrooms and cook for 5 minutes more.

- Add the kale, salt, pepper, thyme, lemon zest and juice, stir, cook for 5 minutes more and take off the heat.

- Stuff the eggplant halves with the mushroom mix. Place them in the oven and bake 400 degrees F for 20 minutes.

- Divide the eggplants between plates, sprinkle parsley and the yogurt on top and serve for lunch.

Nutrition: calories 512, fat 16.4, fiber 17.5, carbs 78, protein 17.2

Delicious Roasted Duck

Preparation Time: 10 minutes

Cooking Time: 4 hours and 50 minutes

Servings: 4

Ingredients:

1 medium duck

1 celery stalk, chopped

2 yellow onions, chopped

2 teaspoons thyme, dried

8 garlic cloves, minced

2 bay leaves

¼ cup parsley, chopped

pinch of salt and black pepper

1 teaspoon herbs de Provence

For the sauce:

1 tablespoon tomato paste

1 yellow onion, chopped

½ teaspoon sugar

½ cup white wine

3 cups water

1 cup chicken stock

1 and ½ cups black olives, pitted and chopped

¼ teaspoon herbs de Provence

Directions:

- In a baking dish, arrange thyme, parsley, garlic and 2 onions. Add duck, season with salt, 1 teaspoon herbs de Provence and pepper.

- Place in the oven at 475 degrees F and roast for 10 minutes. Cover the dish, reduce heat to 275 degrees F and roast duck for 3 hours and 30 minutes.

- Meanwhile, heat a pan over medium heat, add 1 yellow onion, stir and cook for 10 minutes.

- Add tomato paste, stock, sugar, ¼ teaspoon herbs de Provence, olives and water, cover, reduce heat to low and cook for 1 hour.

- Transfer duck to a work surface, carve, discard bones and divide between plates.

- Drizzle the sauce all over and serve right away.

Nutrition: Calories 254 Fat 3 Fiber 3 Carbs 8 Protein 13

Duck Breast with Apricot Sauce

Preparation Time: 10 minutes

Cooking Time: 20 minutes

Servings: 4

Ingredients:

4 duck breasts, boneless

salt and black pepper to taste

¼ teaspoon cinnamon, ground

¼ teaspoon coriander, ground

5 tablespoons apricot preserves

3 tablespoons chives, chopped

2 tablespoons parsley, chopped

drizzle of olive oil

3 tablespoons apple cider vinegar

2 tablespoons red onions, chopped

1 cup apricots, chopped

¾ cup blackberries

Directions:

- Season duck breasts with salt, pepper, coriander and cinnamon, place on a preheated grill pan over medium-high heat, cook for 2 minutes, flip and cook for 3 minutes more.

- Flip duck breasts again, add 3 tablespoons apricot preserves, cook for 1 minute, transfer them to a cutting board, set aside for 2-3 minutes and slice.

- Heat a pan over medium heat, add vinegar, onion, 2 tablespoons apricot preserves, apricots, blackberries, and chives, stir and cook for 3 minutes.

- Divide sliced duck breasts between plates and serve with apricot sauce drizzled on top.

Nutrition: Calories 275 Fat 4 Fiber 4 Carbs 7 Protein 12

Mediterranean Duck Breast Salad

Preparation Time: 10 minutes

Cooking Time: 20 minutes

Servings: 4

Ingredients:

3 tablespoons white wine vinegar

2 tablespoons sugar

2 oranges, peeled and cut into segments

1 teaspoon orange zest, grated

1 tablespoon lemon juice

1 teaspoon lemon zest, grated

3 tablespoons shallot, minced

tablespoons canola oil

salt and black pepper to taste

2 duck breasts, boneless but the skin on, cut into 4 pieces

1 head of frisée, torn

2 small lettuce heads washed, torn into small pieces

2 tablespoons chives, chopped

Directions:

- Heat a small saucepan over medium high heat, add vinegar and sugar, stir and boil for 5 minutes and take off heat.
- Add orange zest, lemon zest and lemon juice, stir and set aside for a few minutes. Add shallot, salt and pepper to taste and the oil, whisk well and set aside for now.
- Pat dry duck pieces, score skin, trim and season with salt and pepper. Heat a pan over medium high heat for 1 minute, arrange duck breast pieces skin side down, brown for 8 minutes, reduce heat to medium and cook for 4 more minutes.
- Flip pieces, cook for 3 minutes, transfer to a cutting board and cover them with foil. Put frisée and lettuce in a bowl, stir and divide between plates.
- Slice duck, arrange on top, add orange segments, sprinkle chives and drizzle the vinaigrette.

Nutrition: Calories 320 Fat 4 Fiber 4 Carbs 6 Protein 14

Duck and Orange Sauce

Preparation Time: 10 minutes

Cooking Time: 5 hours

Servings: 6

Ingredients:

2 medium ducks, fat trimmed

1 tablespoon olive oil

1 cup water

Salt and black pepper to taste

2 tomatoes, chopped

2 carrots, chopped

2 celery stalks, chopped

1 leek, chopped

2 garlic cloves, minced

1 yellow onion, chopped

2 bay leaves

3 tablespoons white flour

1 teaspoon thyme, dried

2 tablespoons tomato paste

1-quart chicken stock

juice of 2 oranges

3 oranges, peeled and cut into segments

1/3 cup sugar

2 tablespoons currant jelly

1/3 cup cider vinegar

2 tablespoons cold butter

Directions:

- Pierce the duck skin, season all over with salt and pepper. Arrange them in a roasting pan, add the water and bake in the oven at 450 degrees F for 20 minutes.

- Reduce heat to 350 degrees F, turn the ducks and bake them for 30 minutes more.

- Turn ducks again and roast them for 30 minutes more. Meanwhile, heat a pan with the oil over high heat, add carrots, celery, leek, tomatoes, garlic, onion, thyme and bay leaves, stir and cook for 10 minutes.

- Add tomato paste, flour, the wine, and the stock gradually, bring to a boil, reduce heat to medium-low, simmer for 50 minutes, take off heat and strain the sauce into a bowl.

- Heat a small pan over medium-high heat, add vinegar and sugar, stir and cook for 4 minutes.

- Add orange juice and currant jelly, stir and bring to a boil. Add strained sauce, salt, and pepper, stir and cook for 8 minutes.

- Add butter gradually and stir well again. Take ducks out of the oven, turn them, place them in the oven again, and cook for 40 more minutes.

- Take ducks out of the oven again, place them under preheated broiler and broil them for 3 minutes.

- Transfer ducks to a platter and keep them warm.

- Heat up juices from the pan in a saucepan over medium heat, take off heat and strain them into a bowl.

- Add this to orange sauce and stir. Arrange the orange segments next to the ducks, and serve with orange sauce.

Nutrition: Calories 342 Fat 13 Fiber 4 Carbs 17 Protein 12

Duck Breast and Blackberries Mix

Preparation Time: 10 minutes

Cooking Time: 25 minutes

Servings: 4

Ingredients:

4 duck breasts

2 tablespoons balsamic vinegar

3 tablespoons sugar

salt and black pepper to taste

1 ½ cups water

4 ounces blackberries

¼ cup chicken stock

1 tablespoon butter

2 teaspoons corn flour

Directions:

- Pat dry duck breasts with paper towels, score the skin, season with salt and pepper to taste and set aside for 30 minutes.

- Put breasts skin side down in a pan, heat over medium heat and cook for 8 minutes.

- Flip breasts and cook for 30 more seconds. Transfer duck breasts to a baking dish skin side up, place in the oven at 425 degrees F and bake for 15 minutes.

- Take the meat out of the oven and set aside to cool down for 10 minutes before you cut them.

- Meanwhile, put sugar in a pan, heat over medium heat and melt it, stirring all the time. Take pan off heat, add the water, stock, balsamic vinegar and the blackberries.

- Heat this mix to medium temperature and cook until sauce is reduced to half. Transfer sauce to another pan, add corn flour mixed with water, heat again and cook for 4 minutes until it thickens.

- Add salt and pepper, the butter and whisk really well.

- Slice the duck breasts, divide between plates and serve with the berries sauce on top.

Nutrition: Calories 320 Fat 15 Fiber 5 Carbs 16 Protein 11

Slow Cooked Mediterranean Duck

Preparation Time: 10 minutes

Cooking Time: 5 hours

Servings: 4

Ingredients:

1 duck, cut into pieces

2 yellow onions, chopped

1 celery rib, chopped

6 garlic cloves, minced

1 and ½ tablespoons thyme, chopped

¼ cup parsley, chopped

pinch of salt and black pepper

½ cup white wine

½ teaspoon sugar

1 cup chicken stock

1 and ½ cups black olives, pitted and sliced

¼ teaspoon Italian seasoning

Directions:

- In a slow cooker, mix the duck with the onions, celery, garlic, thyme, parsley, salt, pepper, wine, sugar, stock, black olives and Italian seasoning.

- Toss, cover and cook on high for 5 hours.

- Divide the duck pieces and the cooking juices between plates and serve.

Nutrition: Calories 320 Fat 14 Fiber 4 Carbs 15 Protein 11

Salmon Bowls

Preparation Time: 10 minutes

Cooking Time: 40 minutes

Servings: 4

Ingredients:

2 cups farro

Juice of 2 lemons

1/3 cup olive oil+ 2 tablespoons

Salt and black pepper

1 cucumber, chopped

¼ cup balsamic vinegar

1 garlic cloves, minced

¼ cup parsley, chopped

¼ cup mint, chopped

2 tablespoons mustard

4 salmon fillets, boneless

Directions:

- Put water in a large pot, bring to a boil over medium-high heat, add salt and the farro, stir, simmer for 30 minutes, drain, transfer to a bowl, add the lemon juice, mustard, garlic, salt, pepper and 1/3 cup oil, toss and set aside for now.

- In another bowl, mash the cucumber with a fork, add the vinegar, salt, pepper, the parsley, dill and mint and whisk well.

- Heat a pan with the rest of the oil over medium heat, add the salmon fillets skin side down, cook for 5 minutes on each side, cool them down and break into pieces.

- Add over the farro, add the cucumber dressing, toss and serve for lunch.

Nutrition: calories 281, fat 12.7, fiber 1.7, carbs 5.8, protein 36.5

Spicy Potato Salad

Preparation Time: 10 minutes

Cooking Time: 15 minutes

Servings: 4

Ingredients:

1 and ½ pounds baby potatoes, peeled and halved

pinch of salt and black pepper

2 tablespoons harissa paste

6 ounces Greek yogurt

juice of 1 lemon

¼ cup red onion, chopped

¼ cup parsley, chopped

Directions:

- Put the potatoes in a pot, add water to cover, add salt, bring to a boil over medium-high heat, cook for 12 minutes, drain and transfer them to a bowl.
- Add the harissa and the rest of the ingredients, toss and serve for lunch.

Nutrition: calories 354, fat 19.2, fiber 4.5, carbs 24.7, protein 11.2

Chicken and Rice Soup

Preparation Time: 10 minutes

Cooking Time: 35 minutes

Servings: 4

Ingredients:

6 cups chicken stock

1 and ½ cups chicken meat, cooked and shredded

1 bay leaf

1 yellow onion, chopped

2 tablespoons olive oil

1/3 cup white rice

1 egg, whisked

juice of ½ lemon

1 cup asparagus, trimmed and halved

1 cup carrots, chopped

½ cup dill, chopped

salt and black pepper to taste

Directions:

- Heat a pot with the oil over medium heat, add the onions and sauté for 5 minutes.
- Add the stock, dill, the rice and the bay leaf, stir, bring to a boil over medium heat and cook for 10 minutes.
- Add the rest of the ingredients except the egg and the lemon juice, stir and cook for 15 minutes more.
- Add the egg whisked with the lemon juice gradually, whisk the soup, cook for 2 minutes more, divide into bowls and serve.

Nutrition: calories 263, fat 18.5, fiber 4.5, carbs 19.8, protein 14.5

Fish Soup

Preparation Time: 10 minutes

Cooking Time: 20 minutes

Servings: 4

Ingredients:

2 tablespoons olive oil

1 tablespoon garlic, minced

½ cup tomatoes, crushed

1 yellow onion, chopped

1 quart veggie stock

1 pound cod, skinless, boneless and cubed

¼ teaspoon rosemary, dried

pinch of salt and black pepper

Directions:

- Heat a pot with the oil over medium heat, add the onion and the garlic and sauté for 5 minutes.

- Add the rest of the ingredients, toss, simmer over medium heat for 15 minutes more, divide into bowls and serve for lunch.

Nutrition: calories 198, fat 8.1, fiber 1, carbs 4.2, protein 26.4

Lamb and Potatoes Stew

Preparation Time: 10 minutes

Cooking Time: 1 hour and 20 minutes

Servings: 4

Ingredients:

2 pounds lamb shoulder, boneless and cubed

salt and black pepper to taste

1 yellow onion, chopped

3 tablespoons olive oil

3 tomatoes, grated

2 cups chicken stock

2 and ½ pounds gold potatoes, cubed

¾ cup green olives, pitted and sliced

1 tablespoon cilantro, chopped

Directions:

- Heat a pot with the oil over medium-high heat, add the lamb, and brown for 5 minutes on each side.

- Add the onion and sauté for 5 minutes more.

- Add the rest of the ingredients, bring to a simmer and cook over medium heat for 1 hour and 10 minutes.

- Divide the stew into bowls and serve.

Nutrition: calories 411, fat 17.4, fiber 8.4, carbs 25.5, protein 34.3

Ground Pork and Tomatoes Soup

Preparation Time: 10 minutes

Cooking Time: 40 minutes

Servings: 4

Ingredients:

1 pound pork meat, ground

salt and black pepper to taste

2 garlic cloves, minced

2 teaspoons thyme, dried

2 tablespoons olive oil

4 cups beef stock

pinch of saffron powder

15 ounces canned tomatoes, crushed

1 tablespoons parsley, chopped

Directions:

- Heat a pot with the oil over medium heat, add the meat and the garlic and brown for 5 minutes.

- Add the rest of the ingredients except the parsley, bring to a simmer and cook for 25 minutes.

- Divide the soup into bowls, sprinkle the parsley on top and serve.

Nutrition: calories 372, fat 17.3, fiber 5.5, carbs 28.4, protein 17.4

Melitzanes Imam/Greek Eggplant Dish

Preparation Time: 30 minutes

Cooking Time: 1 hour 15 minutes

Servings: 2

Ingredients:

eggplant (1)

diced tomatoes, drained (14.5 oz. can)

tomato paste (1 tbsp.)

medium onion (1)

minced garlic (1 tbsp./to taste)

ground cinnamon (1 tsp.)

pepper & salt (as desired)

olive oil (3 tbsp.)

Directions:

- Set the oven to 350° Fahrenheit.

- Slice the eggplant lengthwise in half. Cut out the halves leaving about a one-inch shell. Set the flesh aside.

- Arrange the shells on a baking pan. Lightly spritz the eggplant using oil and bake until softened (30 min.).

- Chop the leftover eggplant into small pieces.

- Prepare a skillet using the medium temperature setting with two tablespoons of oil.

- Dice and add the onion, garlic, and chopped eggplant to sauté for a few minutes.

- Dump in the tomato paste and tomatoes and simmer using the low-heat temperature setting.

- Transfer the shells to the countertop, and spoon in the tomato/eggplant mixture.

- Sprinkle using cinnamon and bake for another 30 minutes and serve.

Nutrition: Calories: 314 Protein: 5.3 grams Fat: 20.8 grams

Red Mediterranean Potato Salad

Preparation Time: 15 minutes

Cooking Time: 25 minutes

Servings: 12

Ingredients:

red potatoes (1.5 lb. - halved)

bacon (3 slices)

grape tomatoes - red/yellow (.75 cup)

chopped onion (.25 cup)

sliced olives (.25 cup)

fat-free Italian dressing (.5 cup)

cider vinegar (1 tbsp.)

Italian parsley (1 tbsp.)

Also needed: 3-quart saucepan

Directions:

- Pour about one inch of water into the pan and let boil.

- Slice and toss in the potatoes. Place a lid on the pot and cook them using the medium temperature setting for 10-15 minutes until tender. Drain and slightly cool.

- Slice the halved potatoes into .75-inch cubes and toss them into a salad dish.

- Prepare a microwave-safe platter with a layer of paper towels. Add in the bacon and cook on high for two to three minutes. Crumble them.

- Stir the tomatoes, bacon, onion, and olives in with the potatoes.

- Whisk the vinegar and dressing. Pour over the potatoes and gently toss.

- Chop the parsley to sprinkle the salad, and serve or chill.

Nutrition: Fat: 1.5 grams Protein: 2 grams Calories: 60

Savory Mediterranean Orzo

Preparation Time: 15 minutes

Cooking Time: 45 minutes

Servings: 12

Ingredients:

chicken broth - reduced sodium (4 cups)

orzo pasta (16 oz. pkg.)

medium onion (1)

olive oil (2 tbsp.)

garlic (4 cloves)

crumbled feta cheese - divided (8 oz./2 cups)

roasted sweet red peppers (7.5 oz. jar)

frozen chopped spinach (10 oz. pkg.)

yellow summer squash (1 small - finely chopped)

salt and black pepper (.5 tsp. each)

Also needed: 13 by 9-inch baking dish

Directions:

- Grease the baking dish and set it to the side for now.

- Pour water into a large saucepan and wait for it to boil. Stir in orzo; cook over medium heat until tender (six to eight minutes). Place the pan on the countertop, off the burner.

- Prepare a pan with oil. Dice and sauté the onion until tender. Mince and add the garlic, sautéing it for one minute longer.

- Drain and chop the jarred peppers. Thaw and squeeze the spinach to remove the liquids. Stir one cup of cheese, squash, red peppers, spinach, salt, and pepper into the orzo mixture.

- Place the mixture into the baking dish, sprinkle it with the rest of the cheese. Bake it without the lid, at 350° Fahrenheit for 20 to 25 minutes until it's thoroughly heated.

Nutrition: Fat: 6 grams Protein: 10 grams Calories: 233

Spinach Pie

Preparation Time: 20 minutes

Cooking Time: 60 minutes

Servings: 6

Ingredients:

melted butter (.5 cup)

frozen spinach (10 oz. pkg.)

fresh parsley (.5 cup)

green onions (.5 cup)

fresh dill (.5 cup)

crumbled feta cheese (.5 cup)

cream cheese (4 oz.)

cottage cheese (4 oz.)

Parmesan (2 tbsp. - grated)

large eggs (2)

pepper and salt (as desired)

phyllo dough (40 sheets)

Directions:

- Heat the oven to 350° Fahrenheit.

- Mince/chop the onions, dill, and parsley. Thaw spinach and sheets of dough. Dab spinach dry by squeezing.

- Combine the spinach, scallions, eggs, cheeses, parsley, dill, pepper, and salt in a blender until creamy.

- Prepare the small phyllo triangles by filling them with one teaspoon of the spinach mixture.

- Lightly brush the outside of the triangles with butter and arrange them with the seam-side facing downwards on an ungreased baking tray.

- Place them in the heated oven to bake until golden brown and puffed (20-25 min.). Serve piping hot.

Nutrition: Calories: 555 Protein: 18.7 grams Fat: 21.3 grams

Cannellini Bean Lettuce Wraps

Preparation Time: 10 minutes

Cooking Time: 15 minutes

Servings: 4

Ingredients:

Olive oil (1 tbsp.)

red onion (.5 cup)

tomatoes (1 medium/.75 cup)

freshly cracked black pepper (.25 tsp.)

fresh curly parsley (.25 cup)

great northern beans or cannellini beans (15 oz. can)

prepared hummus (.5 cup)

Romaine lettuce leaves (8)

Directions:

- Drain and rinse the vegetables and beans. Chop the tomatoes and onion into fine pieces.

- Add the oil into a skillet at medium heat.

- Chop and toss in the onions, tomatoes, and pepper and sauté. Stir occasionally.

- Pour in the drained beans and simmer them for three additional minutes.

- Mix in the parsley after removing it from the burner.

- Spread the hummus over each of the leaves of lettuce. Spread the bean mixture to the center of each leaf. Fold it over to make a wrap and serve.

Nutrition: Calories: 235 Protein: 4 grams Fat: 20 grams

Easy Farfalle with Fresh Tomatoes

Preparation Time: 15 minutes

Cooking Time: 25-30 minutes

Servings: 4

Ingredients:

tomatoes (4/2 lb. total weight)

fresh basil (.5 cup)

red onion (3 tbsp.)

garlic (1 clove)

olive oil (3 tbsp.)

red wine vinegar (1 tbsp.)

black pepper (.25 tsp.)

salt (.75 tsp.)

farfalle pasta (.5 lb.)

Directions:

- Peel and remove seeds from the tomatoes and dice into ½-inch pieces. Cut basil into slender ribbons, using the whole leaves for garnishing. Chop/mince the garlic and onion.

- Prepare the sauce in a large mixing container using the tomatoes, onion, basil oil, garlic, vinegar, pepper, and salt. Toss to mix.

- Prepare a large pot of water (about ¾ full) and wait for it to boil. Toss in the farfalle and simmer until it's al dente (10 min.) Pour it into a colander to drain.

- Divide the pasta and sauce between the bowls and serve.

Nutrition: Calories: 212.5 Protein: 4.2 grams Fat: 11.2 grams

Fried Rice with Spinach - Peppers & Artichokes

Preparation Time: 10 minutes

Cooking Time: 15-20 minutes

Servings: 4

Ingredients:

cooked rice (1.5 cups)

frozen chopped spinach (10 oz.)

marinated artichoke hearts (6 oz.)

roasted red peppers (4 oz.)

minced garlic (.5 tsp.)

crumbled feta cheese with herbs (.5 cup)

olive oil (2 tbsp.)

Directions:

- Prepare the vegetables. Mince the garlic. Thaw and drain the frozen spinach. Drain and quarter the artichoke hearts. Drain and chop the roasted red peppers.

- Heat a skillet on the stovetop to warm the oil using the medium heat setting. Toss in the garlic to sauté for two minutes.

- Toss in the rice and continue cooking for about two minutes until well heated.

- Fold in the spinach and continue cooking for three more minutes.

- Add the red peppers and artichoke hearts. Simmer for two minutes.

- Stir in the feta cheese and serve immediately.

Nutrition: Calories: 244 Protein: 9.3 grams Fat: 12.9 grams

Gigantes (Greek Lima Beans)

Preparation Time: 1 hour

Cooking Time: 10 hours

Servings: 8

Ingredients:

dried lima beans (16 oz. pkg.)

chopped tomatoes with juice (2 - 16 oz. cans)

olive oil (1 cup)

minced garlic (3 cloves)

sea salt (as desired)

freshly chopped dill (1 tsp.)

Also needed: 9 x 13 baking dish

Directions:

- Pour the beans into a large saucepan with water to fill two inches over the top of the beans. Set them aside to soak overnight.

- Set the oven to 375° Fahrenheit.

- Place the saucepan over medium heat and wait for it to boil. Once it's boiling, lower the temperature to med-low and simmer for 20 minutes. Dump out the water and drain the beans in a colander.

- Fold the beans into the baking dish with the dill, salt, oil, garlic, and tomatoes.

- Bake the beans for 1.5 to 2 hours. Add water as needed, stirring occasionally.

Nutrition: Calories: 449 Protein: 13 grams Fat: 27.5 grams

Gluten-Free Spanish Rice

Preparation Time: 15 minutes

Cooking Time: 40 minutes

Servings: 6

Ingredients:

olive oil (1 tbsp.)

garlic (2 cloves)

medium onion (.5 cup)

medium green bell pepper (.5 cup)

long-grain rice - regular/uncooked (1 cup)

sea salt (.25 tsp.)

crushed red pepper (.25 tsp.)

chicken broth (1.75 cups)

undrained - diced fire-roasted tomatoes (1 - 14.5 oz. can)

Also needed: 3-quart saucepan

Directions:

- Heat the oil in the saucepan using the medium temperature setting.

- Chop/dice the onion, garlic, and bell pepper and toss into the skillet for about five minutes, stirring constantly.

- Add in red pepper, salt, broth (reduced-sodium is best), rice, and tomatoes. Wait for it to boil. Reduce the temperature setting and cook until the rice is tender before serving (20-25 min.).

Nutrition: Calories: 170 Protein: 4 grams Fat: 2.5 grams

Chapter 4:
Dinner

Spaghetti in Clam Sauce

Preparation Time:5 minutes

Cooking Time:45 minutes

Servings: 4

Ingredients:

8 oz. spaghetti

2 tablespoons olive oil

2 garlic cloves, minced

2 tomatoes, peeled and diced

1 cup cherry tomatoes, halved

1-pound fresh clams, cleaned and rinsed

2 tablespoons white wine

1 teaspoon sherry vinegar

Directions:

- Heat oil in a heavy saucepan and add the garlic. Cook for 30 seconds until fragrant, then add the tomatoes, wine and vinegar.

- Bring to a boil and cook for 5 minutes; stir in the clams and continue cooking for 10 more minutes.

- In the meantime, bring a large pot of water to a boil with a pinch of salt and add the spaghetti.

- Cook for 8 minutes until al dente. Drain well and mix with the clam sauce.

- Serve the dish right away.

Nutrition: Calories:305, Fat:8.8g, Protein:8.1g, Carbohydrates:48.3g

Creamy Fish Gratin

Preparation Time:5 minutes

Cooking Time:1 hour

Servings: 6

Ingredients:

1 cup heavy cream

2 salmon fillets, cubed

2 cod fillets, cubed

2 sea bass fillets, cubed

1 celery stalk, sliced

salt and pepper to taste

½ cup grated Parmesan

½ cup feta cheese, crumbled

Directions:

- Combine the cream with the fish fillets and celery in a deep-dish baking pan.
- Add salt and pepper to taste then top with Parmesan and feta cheese.
- Cook in the preheated oven at 350F for 20 minutes.
- Serve the gratin right away.

Nutrition: Calories:301, Fat:16.1g, Protein:36.9g, Carbohydrates:1.3g

Broccoli Pesto Spaghetti

Preparation Time:5 minutes

Cooking Time:35 minutes

Servings: 4

Ingredients:

8 oz. spaghetti

1-pound broccoli, cut into florets

2 tablespoons olive oil

4 garlic cloves, chopped

4 basil leaves

2 tablespoons blanched almonds

1 lemon, juiced

salt and pepper to taste

Directions:

- For the pesto, combine the broccoli, oil, garlic, basil, lemon juice and almonds in a blender and pulse until well mixed and smooth.

- Cook the spaghetti in a large pot of salty water for 8 minutes or until al dente. Drain well.

- Mix the warm spaghetti with the broccoli pesto and serve right away.

Nutrition: Calories:284, Fat:10.2g, Protein:10.4g, Carbohydrates:40.2g

Spaghetti all'Olio

Preparation Time:5 minutes

Cooking Time:30 minutes

Servings: 4

Ingredients:

8 oz. spaghetti

3 tablespoons olive oil

4 garlic cloves, minced

2 red peppers, sliced

1 tablespoon lemon juice

salt and pepper to taste

½ cup grated parmesan cheese

Directions:

- Heat the oil in a skillet and add the garlic. Cook for 30 seconds then stir in the red peppers and cook for 1 more minute on low heat, making sure to only infuse them, not to burn or fry them.

- Add the lemon juice and remove from heat.

- Cook the spaghetti in a large pot of salty water for 8 minutes or as stated on the package, just until al dente.

- Drain the spaghetti well and mix them with the garlic and pepper oil.

- Serve right away.

Nutrition: Calories:268, Fat:11.9g, Protein:7.1g, Carbohydrates:34.1g

Quick Tomato Spaghetti

Preparation Time:5 minutes

Cooking Time:15 minutes

Servings: 4

Ingredients:

8 oz. spaghetti

3 tablespoons olive oil

4 garlic cloves, sliced

1 jalapeno, sliced

2 cups cherry tomatoes

salt and pepper to taste

1 teaspoon balsamic vinegar

½ cup grated Parmesan

Directions:

- Heat a large pot of water on medium flame. Add a pinch of salt and bring to a boil then add the pasta.
- Cook for 8 minutes or until al dente.
- While the pasta cooks, heat oil in a skillet and add the garlic and jalapeno. Cook for 1 minute, then stir in the tomatoes, as well as salt and pepper.
- Cook for 5-7 minutes until the tomato skins burst.
- Add the vinegar and remove from heat.
- Drain the pasta well and mix with the tomato sauce.
- Sprinkle with cheese and serve right away.

Nutrition: Calories:298, Fat:13.5g, Protein:9.7g, Carbohydrates:36.0g

---

Creamy Chicken Soup

Preparation Time: 10 minutes

Cooking Time: 1 hour

Servings: 8

Ingredients:

2 cups eggplant, cubed

salt and black pepper to taste

¼ cup olive oil

1 yellow onion, chopped

2 tablespoons garlic, minced

1 red bell pepper, chopped

2 tablespoons hot paprika

¼ cup parsley, chopped

1 and ½ tablespoons oregano, chopped

4 cups chicken stock

1 pound chicken breast, skinless, boneless and cubed

1 cup half and half

2 egg yolks

¼ cup lime juice

Directions:

- Heat a pot with the oil over medium heat, add the chicken, garlic and onion, and brown for 10 minutes.

- Add the bell pepper and the rest of the ingredients except the half and half, egg, yolks and the lime juice

- Bring to a simmer and cook over medium heat for 40 minutes.

- In a bowl, combine the egg yolks with the remaining ingredients with 1 cup of soup, whisk well and pour into pot.

- Whisk the soup, cook for 5 minutes more, divide into bowls and serve.

Nutrition: calories 312, fat 17.4, fiber 5.6, carbs 20.2, protein 15.3

Barley and Chicken Soup

Preparation Time: 10 minutes

Cooking Time: 50 minutes

Servings: 6

Ingredients:

1 pound chicken breasts, skinless, boneless and cubed

1 tablespoon olive oil

salt and black pepper to taste

2 celery stalks, chopped

2 carrots, chopped

1 red onion, chopped

6 cups chicken stock

½ cup parsley, chopped

½ cup barley

1 teaspoon lime juice

Directions:

- Heat a pot with the oil over medium high heat, add the chicken, season with salt and pepper, and brown for cook for 8 minutes.

- Add the onion, carrots and the celery, stir and cook for 3 minutes more.

- Add the rest of the ingredients except the parsley, bring to a boil and simmer over medium heat for 40 minutes.

- Add the parsley, stir, divide the soup into bowls and serve.

Nutrition: calories 311, fat 8.4, fiber 8.3, carbs 17.4, protein 22.3

Chili Oregano Baked Cheese

Preparation Time:5 minutes

Cooking Time:35 minutes

Servings: 4

Ingredients:

8 oz. feta cheese

4 oz. mozzarella, crumbled

1 chili pepper, sliced

1 teaspoon dried oregano

2 tablespoons olive oil

Directions:

- Place the feta cheese in a small deep-dish baking pan.
- Top with the mozzarella then season with pepper slices and oregano.
- Cover the pan with aluminum foil and cook in preheated oven at 350F for 20 minutes.
- Serve the cheese right away.

Nutrition: Calories:292, Fat:24.2g, Protein:16.2g, Carbohydrates:3.7g

Braised Chicken & Artichoke Hearts

Preparation Time: 30 minutes

Cooking Time: 1.5 hours

Servings: 4

Ingredients:

olive oil (1 tbsp.)

chicken legs (4 quarters)

yellow onion (1)

garlic (4 cloves)

black pepper (1 tbsp.)

salt (1 tsp.)

red pepper flakes (.5 tsp.)

chicken stock/low-sodium broth (1-quart)

canned artichoke hearts (10)

cherry peppers (2 cups)

lemons (2 juiced)

fresh thyme (8 sprigs)

butter beans (16 oz. can)

Also needed: Dutch oven

Directions:

- Dice the onion and garlic. Drain the butter beans. Drain the artichokes and cut them in half.

- Heat the oven to 375° Fahrenheit.

- Prepare pan using the high-temperature setting and add the oil.

- Sear the chicken until browned or about five minutes per side. Set aside on a warm platter.

- Mix in the garlic, onion, pepper flakes, salt, and black pepper. Sauté it for about one minute. Stir in the broth and simmer for about a minute. Take the pan off the burner.

- Add the chicken back in the Dutch oven, adding the thyme, lemon juice, cherry peppers, and artichoke hearts.

- Place the skillet in the oven to bake for about one hour.

- Take the chicken out of the cooker and place on a warm platter again.

- Stir the beans into the pan with broth and artichoke mixture.

- Place each leg quarter in a serving dish. Add a ladle of the artichoke, bean, and broth mixture over each serving.

Nutrition: Calories: 707 Protein: 67.9 grams Fat: 34.9 grams

Chicken Thighs with Shallots in Red Wine Vinegar

Preparation Time: 20 minutes

Cooking Time: 35 minutes

Servings: 4

Ingredients:

chicken thighs (32 oz. / 8 lean)

kosher salt and fresh pepper (as desired)

Chicken broth (1 cup)

Red wine vinegar (.5 cup)

honey (1 tbsp.)

butter (1 tsp.)

tomato paste (1 tbsp.)

shallot (1 large or .75 cup)

garlic (2 cloves)

light sour cream (2 tbsp.)

dry white wine (.5 cup)

fresh parsley (2 tbsp.)

Directions:

- Trim the thighs and sprinkle with pepper and salt.

- Prepare a medium saucepan with the honey, ¾ cup of the chicken broth, vinegar, and tomato paste. Boil until it's about ¾ cup (about 5 min.). Take the saucepan off the burner.

- Prepare a large skillet using the med-low temperature setting. Melt the butter and add the chicken. Cook for about six to eight minutes. Remove and set it aside.

- Thinly slice/toss the garlic and shallots into the pan. Sauté for five minutes.

- Pour the sauce, wine, and broth over the chicken. Place a lid on the skillet, and simmer until tender (about 20 min.).

- Remove the chicken and stir in the sour cream. Stir into the sauce and boil a couple of minutes.

- Return the chicken to the skillet and garnish with parsley.

Nutrition: Calories: 353.5 Protein: 46 grams Fat: 11.5 grams

Feta Chicken Burgers

Preparation Time: 15 minutes

Cooking Time: 30 minutes

Servings: 6

Ingredients:

reduced-fat mayonnaise (.25 cup)

finely chopped cucumber (.25 cup)

black pepper (.25 tsp.)

garlic powder (1 tsp.)

chopped roasted sweet red pepper (.5 cup)

Greek seasoning (.5 tsp.)

lean ground chicken (1.5 lb.)

crumbled feta cheese (1 cup)

whole wheat burger buns (6 toasted)

Directions:

- Heat the broiler in the oven ahead of time. Combine the mayo and cucumber. Set aside.

- Whisk each of the seasonings and the red pepper for the burgers. Work in the chicken and the cheese. Shape the mixture into six ½-inch thick patties.

- Broil the burgers approximately four inches from the heat source. It should take about three to four minutes per side until the thermometer reaches 165° Fahrenheit.

- Serve on the buns with the cucumber sauce. Top off with tomato and lettuce if desired and serve.

Nutrition: Calories: 356 Protein: 31 grams Fat: 14 grams

Grecian Chicken & Pasta Skillet

Preparation Time: 15 minutes

Cooking Time: 40 minutes

Servings: 4

Ingredients:

diced tomatoes undrained - no-salt-added (14.5 oz.)

chicken broth - reduced-sodium (14.5 oz.)

chicken breast - cut into 1-inch pieces (.75 lb.)

water or white wine (.5 cup)

garlic (1 clove)

dried oregano (.5 tsp.)

multigrain thin spaghetti (4 oz.)

marinated and quartered artichoke hearts (7.5 oz. jar)

roasted sweet bell pepper strips (.25 cup)

sliced ripe olives (.25 cup)

baby spinach (2 cups)

chopped green onion (1)

fresh parsley (2 tbsp.)

olive oil (1 tbsp.)

grated lemon zest (.5 tsp.)

lemon juice (2 tbsp.)

pepper (.5 tsp.)

Optional: crumbled reduced-fat feta cheese (as desired)

Directions:

- Combine the water/wine, chicken broth, chicken, garlic, oregano, and tomatoes in a large skillet. Drain and coarsely chop the artichoke hearts and add to the skillet.

- Toss in the spaghetti and boil for five to seven minutes. Simmer until chicken is no longer pink or raw.

- Stir in the spinach, pepper, oil, parsley, green onion, olives, red peppers, and the juice and zest of lemon.

- Simmer for another two to three minutes or until the spinach is wilted.

- Sprinkle with the cheese and serve.

Nutrition: Calories: 373 Protein: 25 grams Fat: 15 grams

Greek Penne & Chicken

Preparation Time: 20 minutes

Cooking Time: 50 minutes

Servings: 4

Ingredients:

skinless - boneless chicken breast halves (1 lb.)

penne pasta (16 oz. pkg.)

butter (1.5 tbsp.)

salted butter (16 oz.)

red onion (.5 cup)

cloves of garlic (2)

artichoke hearts in water (14 oz.)

tomato (1 chopped)

Hunt's diced tomatoes (14.5 oz.)

Crumbled feta cheese (.5 cup)

fresh parsley (3 tbsp.)

black pepper and salt (as desired)

lemon juice (2 tbsp.)

dried oregano (1 tsp.)

Directions:

- Slice the chicken into bite-sized pieces.

- Prepare the penne until al dente and drain it thoroughly.

- Melt the butter in a skillet using the med-high temperature setting.
- Mince and toss in the garlic and onion. Sauté them for two minutes. Fold in the chicken and continue cooking for another five to six minutes.
- Reduce the temperature to med-low.
- Drain and add the artichoke hearts with the remainder of the ingredients.
- Simmer for about two to three minutes or until hot.
- Chop the parsley and add the salt and pepper to the chicken before serving.

Nutrition: Calories: 685 Protein: 47 grams Fat: 13 grams

Easy and Simple Chicken

Preparation Time: 8 hours and 10 minutes

Cooking Time: 30 minutes

Servings: 8

Ingredients:

whole chicken, cut into medium pieces

pinch of salt and black pepper

½ cup olive oil

1 tablespoon rosemary, chopped

garlic cloves, minced

1 tablespoon thyme, chopped

1 tablespoon oregano, chopped

juice from 2 lemons

Directions:

- In a bowl, mix oil with salt, pepper, garlic, rosemary, thyme, oregano and lemon juice and whisk well.

- Add chicken, toss well and keep in the fridge for 8 hours.

- Place chicken pieces on preheated grill pan over medium heat, cook for 15 minutes on each side.

- divide between plates and serve with a side salad.

Nutrition: Calories 287 Fat 3 Fiber 1 Carbs 4 Protein 20

Dill Relish on White Sea Bass

Preparation Time: 5 minutes

Cooking Time: 12 minutes

Servings: 4

Ingredients:

1 ½ tbsp chopped white onion

1 ½ tsp chopped fresh dill

1 lemon, quartered

1 tsp Dijon mustard

1 tsp lemon juice

1 tsp pickled baby capers, drained

4 pieces of 4-oz white sea bass fillets

Directions:

- Preheat oven to 375oF.

- Mix lemon juice, mustard, dill, capers and onions in a small bowl.

- Prepare four aluminum foil squares and place 1 fillet per foil.

- Squeeze a lemon wedge per fish.

- Evenly divide into 4 the dill spread and drizzle over fillet.

- Place the foil over the fish securely and pop in the oven.

- Bake for 10 to 12 minutes or until fish is cooked through.

Remove from foil and transfer to a serving platter; serve and enjoy.

Nutrition: Calories per Servings: 115 Protein: 7g Fat: 1gCarbs: 12g

Fish and Orzo

Preparation Time: 10 minutes

Cooking Time: 35 minutes

Servings: 4

Ingredients:

1 teaspoon garlic, minced

1 teaspoon red pepper, crushed

2 shallots, chopped

1 tablespoon olive oil

1 teaspoon anchovy paste

1 tablespoon oregano, chopped

2 tablespoons black olives, pitted and chopped

2 tablespoons capers, drained

15 ounces canned tomatoes, crushed

pinch of salt and black pepper

4 cod fillets, boneless

1 ounce feta cheese, crumbled

1 tablespoons parsley, chopped

3 cups chicken stock

1 cup orzo pasta

zest of 1 lemon, grated

Directions:

- Heat a pan with the oil over medium heat, add the garlic, red pepper and the shallots and sauté for 5 minutes.

- Add the anchovy paste, oregano, black olives, capers, tomatoes, salt and pepper, stir and cook for 5 minutes more.

- Add the cod fillets, sprinkle the cheese and the parsley on top, Place in the oven and bake at 375 degrees F for 15 minutes more.

- Meanwhile, put the stock in a pot, bring to a boil over medium heat, add the orzo and the lemon zest, bring to a simmer, cook for 10 minutes, fluff with a fork, and divide between plates.

- Top each serving with the fish mix and serve.

Nutrition: Calories 402 Fat 21 Fiber 8 Carbs 21 Protein 31

Baked Sea Bass

Preparation Time: 10 minutes

Cooking Time: 12 minutes

Servings: 4

Ingredients:

4 sea bass fillets, boneless

salt and black pepper to taste

2 cups potato chips, crushed

1 tablespoon mayonnaise

Directions:

- Season the fish fillets with salt and pepper, brush with the mayonnaise and dredge each in the potato chips.

- Arrange the fillets on a baking sheet lined with parchment paper and bake at 400 degrees F for 12 minutes.

- Divide the fish between plates and serve with a side salad.

Nutrition: Calories 228 Fat 8.6 Fiber 0.6 Carbs 9.3 Protein 25

Fish and Tomato Sauce

Preparation Time: 10 minutes

Cooking Time: 30 minutes

Servings: 4

Ingredients:

4 cod fillets, boneless

2 garlic cloves, minced

2 cups cherry tomatoes, halved

1 cup chicken stock

pinch of salt and black pepper

¼ cup basil, chopped

Directions:

- Put the tomatoes, garlic, salt and pepper in a pan, heat up over medium heat and cook for 5 minutes.
- Add the fish and the rest of the ingredients, bring to a simmer, cover the pan and cook for 25 minutes.
- Divide the mix between plates and serve.

Nutrition: Calories 180 Fat 1.9 Fiber 1.4 Carbs 5.3 Protein 33.8

Halibut and Quinoa Mix

Preparation Time: 10 minutes

Cooking Time: 12 minutes

Servings: 4

Ingredients:

4 halibut fillets, boneless

2 tablespoons olive oil

1 teaspoon rosemary, dried

2 teaspoons cumin, ground

1 tablespoons coriander, ground

2 teaspoons cinnamon powder

2 teaspoons oregano, dried

pinch of salt and black pepper

2 cups quinoa, cooked

1 cup cherry tomatoes, halved

1 avocado, peeled, pitted and sliced

1 cucumber, cubed

½ cup black olives, pitted and sliced

juice of 1 lemon

Directions:

- In a bowl, combine the fish with the rosemary, cumin, coriander, cinnamon, oregano, salt and pepper and toss.

- Heat a pan with the oil over medium heat, add the fish, and sear for 2 minutes on each side.

- Place the pan in the oven and bake the fish at 425 degrees F for 7 minutes.

- Meanwhile, in a bowl, mix the quinoa with the remaining ingredients, toss and divide between plates.

- Add the fish next to the quinoa mix and serve right away.

Nutrition: Calories 364 Fat 15.4 Fiber 11.2 Carbs 56.4 Protein 24.5

Lemon and Dates Barramundi

Preparation Time: 10 minutes

Cooking Time: 12 minutes

Servings: 2

Ingredients:

2 barramundi fillets, boneless

1 shallot, sliced

4 lemon slices

juice of ½ lemon

zest of 1 lemon, grated

2 tablespoons olive oil

6 ounces baby spinach

¼ cup almonds, chopped

4 dates, pitted and chopped

¼ cup parsley, chopped

salt and black pepper to taste

Directions:

- Season fish with salt and pepper and arrange on 2 parchment paper pieces.

- Top fish with the lemon slices, drizzle the lemon juice, and then top with the other ingredients except the oil.

- Drizzle 1 tablespoon oil over each fish mix, wrap the parchment paper around the fish shaping to packets and arrange them on a baking sheet.

- Bake at 400 degrees F for 12 minutes, cool the mix a bit, unfold, divide everything between plates and serve.

Nutrition: Calories 232 Fat 16.5 Fiber 11.1 Carbs 24.8 Protein 6.5

Fish Cakes

Preparation Time: 10 minutes

Cooking Time: 10 minutes

Servings: 6

Ingredients:

20 ounces canned sardines, drained and mashed well

2 garlic cloves, minced

2 tablespoons dill, chopped

1 yellow onion, chopped

1 cup panko breadcrumbs

1 egg, whisked

pinch of salt and black pepper

2 tablespoons lemon juice

5 tablespoons olive oil

Directions:

- In a bowl, combine the sardines with the garlic, dill and the rest of the ingredients except the oil, stir well and shape medium cakes out of this mix.

- Heat a pan with the oil over medium-high heat, add the fish cakes, cook for 5 minutes on each side.

- Serve the cakes with a side salad.

Nutrition: Calories 288 Fat 12.8 Fiber 10.2 Carbs 22.2 Protein 6.8

Baked Salmon with Dill

Preparation Time: 10 minutes

Cooking Time: 15 minutes

Servings: 4

Ingredients:

salmon fillets (4- 6 oz. portions - 1-inch thickness)

kosher salt (.5 tsp.)

finely chopped fresh dill (1.5 tbsp.)

black pepper (.125 tsp.)

lemon wedges (4)

Directions:

- Warm the oven in advance to 350° Fahrenheit.

- Lightly grease a baking sheet with a misting of cooking oil spray and add the fish.

- Lightly spritz the fish with the spray along with a shake of salt, pepper, and dill.

- Bake until the fish is easily flaked (10 min.).

- Serve with lemon wedges.

Nutrition: Calories: 251 Protein: 28 grams Fat: 16 grams

Couscous with Pepperoncini & Tuna

Preparation Time: 10 minutes

Cooking Time: 20 minutes

Servings: 4

Ingredients:

Couscous:

chicken broth or water (1 cup)

couscous (1.25 cups)

kosher salt (.75 tsp.)

The accompaniments:

oil-packed tuna (2- 5-oz. cans)

cherry tomatoes (1 pint - halved)

sliced pepperoncini (.5 cup)

chopped fresh parsley (.33 cup)

capers (.25 cup)

olive oil (for servings)

black pepper and kosher salt to taste

lemon (1 quartered)

Directions:

- Make couscous in a small saucepan using water or broth. Prepare it using the medium heat temperature setting. Let sit for about ten minutes.

- Toss the tomatoes, tuna, capers, parsley, and pepperoncini into a mixing bowl.

- Fluff the couscous when done and dust with pepper and salt. Spritz with oil and serve with the tuna mix and a lemon wedge.

Nutrition: Calories: 226 Protein: 8 grams Fat: 1 gram

Herb-Crusted Halibut

Preparation Time: 10 minutes

Cooking Time: 25 minutes

Servings: 4

Ingredients:

fresh parsley (.33 cup)

fresh dill (.25 cup)

fresh chives (.25 cup)

lemon zest (1 tsp.)

panko breadcrumbs (.75 cup)

olive oil (1 tbsp.)

freshly cracked black pepper (.25 tsp.)

sea salt (1 tsp.)

halibut fillets (4 - 6 oz.)

Directions:

- Chop the fresh dill, chives, and parsley. Prepare a baking tray with a sheet of foil. Set the oven to reach 400° Fahrenheit.

- Combine the salt, pepper, lemon zest, olive oil, chives, dill, parsley, and the breadcrumbs in a mixing bowl.

- Rinse the halibut thoroughly. Use paper towels to dry it before baking.

- Arrange the fish on the baking sheet. Spoon the crumbs over the fish and press it into each of the fillets.

- Bake it until the top is browned and easily flaked or about 10 to 15 minutes.

Nutrition: Calories: 273 Protein: 38 grams Fat: 7 grams

Pan Roasted Chicken and Potatoes

Preparation Time: 10 minutes

Cooking Time: 1 hour

Servings: 8

Ingredients:

3 pounds potatoes, peeled and roughly chopped

2 green bell peppers, chopped

yellow onion, chopped

4 garlic cloves, minced

½ cup black olives, pitted and sliced

14 ounces canned tomatoes, chopped

16 chicken drumsticks, skinless

1 tablespoon mixed herbs, dried

ounces feta cheese, crumbled

½ cup parsley, chopped

Directions:

- Place potatoes in a large saucepan, add water to cover, bring to a boil over medium heat, cook for a couple of minutes, drain and transfer to a large roasting pan.

- Add green bell pepper, onion, garlic, tomatoes, olives and herbs and toss.

- Add chicken, some salt and pepper, toss again, place in the oven at 400 degrees F and roast for 40 minutes.

- Toss everything again and roast for 20 minutes more.

- Divide on plates, sprinkle parsley and feta on top and serve.

Nutrition: Calories 298 Fat 3 Fiber 3 Carbs 7 Protein 16

Crispy Italian Chicken

Preparation Time:5 minutes

Cooking Time:40 minutes

Servings: 4

Ingredients:

4 chicken legs

1 teaspoon dried basil

1 teaspoon dried oregano

salt and pepper to taste

3 tablespoons olive oil

1 tablespoon balsamic vinegar

Directions:

- Season the chicken with salt, pepper, basil and oregano.

- Heat oil in a skillet and add the chicken into the hot oil.

- Cook on each side for 5 minutes until golden then cover the skillet with a weight (another skillet or a very heavy lid is recommended).

- Place over medium heat and cook for 10 minutes on one side, then flip the chicken repeatedly, cooking for another 10 minutes until crispy.

- Serve the chicken right away.

Nutrition: Calories:262, Fat:13.9g, Protein:32.6g, Carbohydrates:0.3g

Sea Bass in a Pocket

Preparation Time:5 minutes

Cooking Time:40 minutes

Servings: 4

Ingredients:

4 sea bass fillets

4 garlic cloves, sliced

1 celery stalk, sliced

1 zucchini, sliced

1 cup cherry tomatoes, halved

1 shallot, sliced

1 teaspoon dried oregano

salt and pepper to taste

Directions:

- Mix garlic, celery, zucchini, tomatoes, shallot and oregano in a bowl. Add salt and pepper to taste.
- Take 4 sheets of baking paper and arrange on your working surface.
- Spoon the vegetable mixture into the center of each sheet.
- Top with a fish fillet then wrap the paper well so it resembles a pocket.
- Place the wrapped fish in a baking tray and cook in the preheated oven at 350F for 15 minutes.
- Serve the fish warm and fresh.

Nutrition: Calories:149, Fat:2.8g, Protein:25.2g, Carbohydrates:5.2g

Chicken and Chorizo Casserole

Preparation Time:5 minutes

Cooking Time:1 hour

Servings: 6

Ingredients:

6 chicken thighs

4 chorizo links, sliced

2 tablespoons olive oil

1 cup tomato juice

2 tablespoons tomato paste

1 bay leaf

1 teaspoon dried thyme

salt and pepper to taste

Directions:

- Heat oil in a skillet and add the chicken. Cook on all sides until golden then transfer the chicken to a deep-dish baking pan.

- Add the rest of the ingredients and season with salt and pepper.

- Cook in the preheated oven at 350F for 25 minutes.

- Serve the casserole right away.

Nutrition: Calories:424, Fat:27.5g, Protein:39.1g, Carbohydrates:3.6g

Lamb Stuffed Tomatoes with Herbs

Preparation Time:5 minutes

Cooking Time:1 hour

Servings: 6

Ingredients:

6 large tomatoes

1-pound ground lamb

¼ cup white rice

2 shallots, chopped

2 garlic cloves, minced

1 tablespoon chopped dill

1 tablespoon chopped parsley

1 tablespoon chopped cilantro

1 teaspoon dried mint

salt and pepper to taste

1 tablespoon lemon juice

2 tablespoons olive oil

1 cup vegetable stock

Directions:

- Mix the lamb, rice, shallots, garlic, dill, parsley, cilantro and mint in a bowl. Add salt and pepper to taste.

- Remove the top of each tomato then carefully remove the flesh, leaving the skins intact.

- Chop the flesh finely and place it in a deep heavy saucepan. Add the lemon juice and salt and pepper to taste.

- Stuff the tomatoes with the lamb mixture and place them all in the pan.

- Drizzle with oil then pour in the stock.

- Cover with a lid and cook on low heat for 35 minutes.

- Serve the tomatoes right away.

Nutrition: Calories:248, Fat:10.7g, Protein:23.7g, Carbohydrates:14.6g

Creamy Spinach with Polenta and Poached Egg

Preparation Time:5 minutes

Cooking Time:40 minutes

Servings: 4

Ingredients:

Creamy spinach:

2 tablespoons olive oil

2 garlic cloves, minced

1 red pepper, chopped

4 cups baby spinach

½ cup heavy cream

1 tablespoon all-purpose flour

salt and pepper to taste

Polenta:

½ cup polenta flour

1 ½ cups water

1 tablespoon olive oil

salt and pepper to taste

Poached eggs:

3 cups water

1 tablespoon white wine vinegar

4 eggs

Directions:

- For the creamy spinach, heat the oil in a skillet and add the garlic and red pepper. Cook on high heat for 1 minute then add the spinach and continue cooking for 5-7 minutes until the spinach is softened and most of the liquid has evaporated.

- Mix the cream with the flour and pour it over the spinach.

- Cook for 5 more minutes until thickened and creamy.

- Adjust the taste with salt and pepper and remove from heat.

- For the polenta, heat the water with salt in a saucepan.

- When it starts to boil, stir in the oil and polenta flour.

- Cook on low heat for 10 minutes.

- For the poached eggs, bring the water, vinegar and a pinch of salt to a boil in a saucepan.

- Crack open the eggs and drop them in the boiling liquid, one by one, cooking them for 1-2 minutes just until set, but still soft in the center.

- To serve, spoon the polenta onto plates. Top with creamy spinach and finish with a poached egg.

Nutrition: Calories:231, Fat:20.7g, Protein:7.3g, Carbohydrates:5.7g

Grilled Vegetable Feta Tart

Preparation Time:5 minutes

Cooking Time:1 ½ hours

Servings: 8

Ingredients:

Crust:

2 cups all-purpose flour

1 teaspoon instant yeast

½ teaspoon salt

1 cup water

2 tablespoons olive oil

Topping:

1 zucchini, sliced

2 tomatoes, sliced

1 shallot, sliced

1 teaspoon dried basil

1 teaspoon dried oregano

2 garlic cloves, minced

2 tablespoons tomato paste

4 oz. feta cheese, crumbled

Directions:

- For the crust, combine all the ingredients in a bowl and mix well. Knead for a few minutes until elastic.

- Allow the dough to rest and rise for 20 minutes, then roll it into a thin round of dough.

- Place the dough on a baking tray.

- Mix the garlic, basil, oregano and tomato paste in a bowl. Spread the mixture over the dough.

- Heat a grill pan over medium flame and place the zucchini and tomatoes on the grill. Cook for a few minutes on all sides until browned.

- Top the tart with the vegetables and shallot, then sprinkle the cheese on top.

- Bake in the preheated oven at 350F for 25 minutes.

- Serve the tart warm and fresh.

Nutrition: Calories:198, Fat:7.0g, Protein:6.3g, Carbohydrates:28.0g

Tomato and Halloumi Platter

Preparation Time: 5 minutes

Cooking Time: 4 minutes

Servings: 4

Ingredients:

1 pound tomatoes, sliced

½ pound halloumi, cut into 4 slices

2 tablespoons parsley, chopped

1 tablespoon basil, chopped

2 tablespoons olive oil

pinch of salt and black pepper

juice of 1 lemon

Directions:

- Brush the halloumi slices with half the oil, put them on a preheated grill and cook over medium-high heat and cook for 2 minutes on each side.

- Arrange the tomato slices on a platter, season with salt and pepper, drizzle the lemon juice and the rest of the oil all over, top with the halloumi slices, sprinkle the herbs on top and serve for lunch.

Nutrition: calories 181, fat 7.3, fiber 1.4, carbs 4.6, protein 1.1

Chickpeas and Millet Stew

Preparation Time: 10 minutes

Cooking Time: 1 hour and 5 minutes

Servings: 4

Ingredients:

1 cup millet

2 tablespoons olive oil

pinch of salt and black pepper

1 eggplant, cubed

1 yellow onion, chopped

14 ounces canned tomatoes, chopped

14 ounces canned chickpeas, drained and rinsed

3 garlic cloves, minced

2 tablespoons harissa paste

1 bunch cilantro, chopped

2 cups water

Directions:

- Put the water in a pan, bring to a simmer over medium heat, add the millet, simmer for 25 minutes, take off the heat, fluff with a fork and set aside for now.

- Heat a pan with half of the oil over medium heat, add the eggplant, salt and pepper, stir, cook for 10 minutes and transfer to a bowl.

- Add the rest of the oil to the pan, heat up over medium heat again, add the onion and sauté for 10 minutes.

- Add the garlic, more salt and pepper, the harrisa, chickpeas, tomatoes and return the eggplant, stir and cook over low heat for 15 minutes more.

- Add the millet, toss, divide the mix into bowls, sprinkle the cilantro on top and serve.

Nutrition: calories 671, fat 15.6, fiber 27.5, carbs 87.5, protein 27.1

Chapter 5:
Snacks

Traditional Mediterranean Hummus

Preparation Time: 10 minutes

Cooking Time: 45 minutes

Servings: 7

Ingredients:

1 cup chickpeas, soaked

6 cups of water

½ cup lemon juice

3 tablespoon olive oil

1 teaspoon salt

1/3 teaspoon harissa

Directions:

- Combine chickpeas and water and boil for 45 minutes or until chickpeas are tender.
- Then transfer chickpeas to the food processor.
- Add 1 cup of chickpeas water and lemon juice.
- Add salt and harissa.
- Blend the hummus until it is smooth and fluffy.
- Add olive oil and pulse it for 10 seconds more.
- Transfer the cooked hummus to the bowl and store in the fridge for up to 2 days.

Nutrition: calories 160, fat 7.9, fiber 5. carbs 17.8, protein 5.7

Tuna Salad in Lettuce Cups

Preparation Time: 10 minutes

Cooking Time: 10 minutes

Servings:6

Ingredients:

4 Romaine lettuce leaves

8 oz tuna fillet

1 teaspoon balsamic vinegar

½ teaspoon olive oil

1 tablespoon fresh dill, chopped

¼ teaspoon salt

¾ teaspoon chili pepper

1 tomato, chopped

¾ cup plain yogurt

Directions:

- Rub the tuna fillet with salt and chili pepper.

- Then drizzle the fish with olive oil.

- Bake tuna for 10 minutes at 365F.

- Chill it a little and chop.

- In the bowl, combine chopped tuna, Plain yogurt, tomato, fresh dill, and balsamic vinegar. Mix well.

- Fill the lettuce leaves with the tuna mixture.

Nutrition: calories 152, fat 11.2, fiber 0.3, carbs 3.4, protein 9

Rice Burgers

Preparation Time: 10 minutes

Cooking Time: 30 minutes

Servings:4

Ingredients:

1/3 cup rice

1 cup of water

½ teaspoon salt

2 tablespoons ricotta cheese

1 egg

¼ cup yellow onion, diced

1 teaspoon sunflower oil

½ teaspoon ground black pepper

1 tablespoon wheat flour, whole grain

Directions:

- Pour water in a pan. Add rice and salt.
- Close the lid and boil rice for 15 minutes or until it will soak all liquid and will be done.
- Meanwhile, heat up oil in the skillet.
- Add diced onion and roast it until golden brown.
- Combine cooked rice with onion.
- Add ground black pepper, wheat flour, and egg.
- Mix up the mixture. It should smooth but not liquid.
- Then make medium size burgers.
- Bake the burgers for 10 minutes at 355F.
- Top the cooked appetizer with ricotta cheese.

Nutrition: calories 104, fat 3, fiber 0.5, carbs 15.1, protein 3.7

Wheatberry Burgers

Preparation Time: 25 minutes

Cooking Time: 15 minutes

Servings:6

Ingredients:

1 cup wheatberry, cooked

2 eggs

¼ cup ground chicken

1 tablespoon wheat flour, whole grain

1 teaspoon Italian seasoning

1 tablespoon olive oil

1 teaspoon salt

Directions:

- In the mixing bowl mix up together wheatberry and ground chicken.
- Crack eggs in the mixture.
- Then add wheat flour, Italian seasoning, and salt.
- Mix the mass with the help of the spoon until homogenous.
- Then make burgers and freeze them in the freezer for 20 minutes.
- Heat up olive oil in the skillet.
- Place frozen burgers in the hot oil and roast them for 4 minutes from each side over the high heat.
- Then cook burgers for 10 minutes more over the medium heat. Flip them onto another side from time to time.

Nutrition: calories 97, fat 5.7, fiber 1.5, carbs 9.2, protein 5.2

Easy Nachos

Preparation Time: 10 minutes

Cooking Time: 10 minutes

Servings:7

Ingredients:

1 cup nachos

1/3 cup Monterey Jack cheese, shredded

2 oz black olives, sliced

2 tomatoes, chopped

Directions:

- Crash the nachos gently and arrange them in the casserole mold in one layer.
- Make the layer of black olives and tomatoes over the nachos. Flatten the ingredients with a spatula if needed.
- Then make the layer of cheese and cover casserole with foil. Secure the edges.
- Bake the nachos for 10 minutes at 365F.
- Then remove the foil from the mold and serve nachos in the casserole mold.

Nutrition: calories 133, fat 8, fiber 2.3, carbs 10.6, protein 5.4

Eggplant Bites

Preparation Time: 15 minutes

Cooking Time: 30 minutes

Servings:8

Ingredients:

2 eggs, beaten

3 oz Parmesan, grated

1 tablespoon coconut flakes

½ teaspoon ground paprika

1 teaspoon salt

2 eggplants, trimmed

Directions:

- Slice the eggplants into the thin circles with a vegetable slicer.

- After this, sprinkle the vegetables with salt and mix up. Leave them for 5-10 minutes.

- Then drain eggplant juice and sprinkle them with ground paprika.

- Mix together coconut flakes and Parmesan.

- Dip every eggplant circle in the egg and then coat in Parmesan mixture.

- Line baking tray with parchment and place eggplants on it.

- Bake the vegetables for 30 minutes at 360F. Flip the eggplants into another side after 12 minutes of cooking.

Nutrition: calories 87, fat 3.9, fiber 5, carbs 8.7, protein 6.2

Peanut Butter Yogurt Dip

Preparation Time: 10 minutes

Cooking Time: 0 minutes

Servings:4

Ingredients:

2 tablespoons peanut butter

1 oz Greek Yogurt

1 teaspoon sesame seeds

½ teaspoon vanilla extract

1 tablespoon honey

Directions:

- Put peanut butter and Greek yogurt in a large bowl.

- Add sesame seeds, vanilla extract, and honey.

- Stir it carefully.

- Store in the fridge until needed.

Nutrition: calories 74, fat 4.5, fiber 0.6, carbs 6.5, protein 2.9

Roasted Chickpeas

Preparation Time: 10 minutes

Cooking Time: 3 hours

Servings:8

Ingredients:

1 cup chickpeas, canned

1 teaspoon salt

½ teaspoon ground coriander

½ teaspoon ground paprika

½ teaspoon dried thyme

¾ teaspoon cayenne pepper

2 tablespoons olive oil

Directions:

- Drain the chickpeas and dry them carefully with a towel.

- Place them on the baking tray.

- Mix up together salt, ground coriander, ground paprika, dried thyme, and cayenne pepper.

- Sprinkle the chickpeas with spices and shake well.

- After this, drizzle them with olive oil. Give them a good shake again.

- Preheat the oven to 375F.

- Place tray with chickpeas in the preheated oven and cook for 35 minutes.

- Flip the chickpeas on another side from time to time.

Nutrition: calories 122, fat 5.1, fiber 4.5, carbs 15.4, protein 4.9

Salty Almonds

Preparation Time: 1 hour 10 minutes

Cooking Time: 15 minutes

Servings:5

Ingredients:

1 cup almonds

3 tablespoons salt

2 cups of water

Directions:

Bring water to boil.

- After this, add 2 tablespoons of salt in water and stir.
- When salt is dissolved, add almonds and let them soak for at least 1 hour.
- Meanwhile, line the tray with baking paper and preheat the oven to 350F.
- Dry the soaked almonds with a paper towel and arrange in one layer on the tray.
- Sprinkle with remaining salt.
- Bake the snack for 15 minutes. Mix from time to time with a spatula or spoon.

Nutrition: calories 110, fat 9.5, fiber 2.4, carbs 4.1, protein 4

Cheesy Artichoke Dip

Preparation Time: 10 minutes

Cooking Time: 10 minutes

Servings:6

Ingredients:

1 cup sour cream

1 cup fresh spinach

4 oz artichoke hearts, drained

1 cup Mozzarella cheese, shredded

1 teaspoon chili flakes

Directions:

- Chop the artichoke hearts into the tiny pieces.

- Put spinach in a blender and blend until smooth.

- Mix together spinach with artichokes. Add sour cream, Mozzarella cheese, and chili flakes. Stir well.

- Transfer mixture to a mold/pan and flatten it.

- Bake the dip for 10 minutes at 360F.

Nutrition: calories 105, fat 8.9, fiber 1.1, carbs 4, protein 3.3

Date and Fig Smoothie

Preparation Time: 5 minutes

Cooking Time: 0 minutes

Servings:1

Ingredients:

1 date, pitted

1 fig, chopped

1 oz Greek yogurt

1/3 cup organic almond milk

1/3 teaspoon ground cardamom

1 teaspoon honey

Directions:

- Place all ingredients in the food processor.

- Blend the mixture until smooth.

- Pour the cooked smoothie into a serving glass.

Nutrition: calories 146, fat 3.1, fiber 2.7, carbs 27.7, protein 4.3

Cucumber Bites with Creamy Avocado

Preparation Time: 10 minutes

Cooking Time: 0 minutes

Servings:5

Ingredients:

1 cucumber

5 cherry tomatoes

2 oz avocado, pitted

¼ teaspoon minced garlic

¼ teaspoon dried basil

¾ teaspoon sour cream

¾ teaspoon lemon juice

Directions:

- Trim the cucumber and slice it on 5 thick slices.

- Churn avocado until you get creamy texture.

- Add minced garlic, dried basil, sour cream, and lemon juice. Mix up well.

- Spread the avocado over the cucumber slices and top with cherry tomatoes.

Nutrition: calories 56, fat 2.7, fiber 2.5, carbs 8.1, protein 1.7

Tomato Finger Sandwich

Preparation Time: 10 minutes

Cooking Time: 0 minutes

Servings:6

Ingredients:

6 corn tortillas

1 tablespoon cream cheese

1 tablespoon ricotta cheese

½ teaspoon minced garlic

1 tablespoon fresh dill, chopped

2 tomatoes, sliced

Directions:

- Cut tortillas into 2 triangles.
- Mix together cream cheese, ricotta cheese, minced garlic, and dill.
- Spread 6 triangles with cream cheese mixture.
- Place sliced tomato on top and cover with remaining tortilla triangles.

Nutrition: calories 71, fat 1.6, fiber 2.1, carbs 12.8, protein 2.3

Parsley Cheese Balls

Preparation Time: 10 minutes

Cooking Time: 1 minute

Servings:6

Ingredients:

1/3 cup cheddar cheese, shredded

1 tablespoon dried dill

1 egg, beaten

½ teaspoon salt

2 tablespoons coconut flakes

3 tablespoons sunflower oil

Directions:

- Mix together shredded cheese with dried dill, salt, and coconut flakes.

- Add egg and stir carefully until homogenous.

- Make small balls from the cheese mixture.

- Heat up sunflower oil in the skillet.

- Place cheese balls in the hot oil and roast them for 10 seconds from each side.

- Dry the cooked cheese balls with a paper towel.

Nutrition: calories 105, fat 10.4, fiber 0.2, carbs 0.7, protein 2.6

Layered Dip

Preparation Time: 10 minutes

Cooking Time: 0 minutes

Servings:12

Ingredients:

½ cup hummus

8 tablespoons tzatziki

1 cup tomatoes, chopped

1 cup cucumbers, chopped

1 teaspoon olive oil

1 tablespoon lemon juice

1/3 cup fresh parsley, chopped

1 jalapeno pepper, chopped

Directions:

- In the mixing bowl mix up together fresh parsley, lemon juice, olive oil, cucumbers, tomatoes, and chopped jalapeno pepper.

- Then make the layer of ½ part of tomato mixture in the casserole dish.

- Top with layer of hummus.

- Then add remaining tomato mixture and flatten it well.

- Top it with tzatziki and flatten well.

- Store dip in the fridge for up to 3 hours.

Nutrition: calories 49, fat 3.6, fiber 1, carbs 3.3, protein 1.1

Grilled Tempeh Sticks

Preparation Time: 5 minutes

Cooking Time: 8 minutes

Servings:6

Ingredients:

11 oz soy tempeh

1 teaspoon olive oil

½ teaspoon ground black pepper

¼ teaspoon garlic powder

Directions:

- Cut soy tempeh into the sticks.

- Sprinkle every tempeh stick with ground black pepper, garlic powder, and olive oil.

- Preheat grill to 375F.

- Place the tempeh sticks in the grill and cook them for 4 minutes from each side. The time of cooking depends on the tempeh sticks size.

- The cooked tempeh sticks will have a light brown color.

Nutrition: calories 88, fat 2.5, fiber 3.6, carbs 10.2, protein 6.5

Sweet Potato Fries

Preparation Time: 10 minutes

Cooking Time: 35 minutes

Servings: 5

Ingredients:

1 teaspoon Zaatar spices

3 sweet potatoes

1 tablespoon dried dill

1 teaspoon salt

3 teaspoons sunflower oil

½ teaspoon paprika

Directions:

- Pour water in the crockpot. Peel the sweet potatoes and cut them into the fries.
- Line the baking tray with parchment.
- Place the layer of the sweet potato in the tray.
- Sprinkle the vegetables with dried dill, salt, and paprika.
- Then sprinkle sweet potatoes with Zaatar and mix up well with the help of the fingertips.
- Sprinkle the sweet potato fries with sunflower oil.
- Preheat the oven to 375F.
- Bake the sweet potato fries for 35 minutes. Stir the fries every 10 minutes.

Nutrition: calories 28, fat 2.9, fiber 0.2, carbs 0.6, protein 0.2

Italian Style Potato Fries

Preparation Time: 10 minutes

Cooking Time: 40 minutes

Servings:4

Ingredients:

1/3 cup baby red potatoes

1 tablespoon Italian seasoning

3 tablespoons canola oil

1 teaspoon turmeric

½ teaspoon of sea salt

½ teaspoon dried rosemary

1 tablespoon dried dill

Directions:

- Cut the red potatoes into the wedges and transfer in the big bowl.
- Sprinkle the vegetables with Italian seasoning, canola oil, turmeric, sea salt, dried rosemary, and dried dill.
- Shake the potato wedges carefully.
- Line the baking tray with baking paper.
- Place the potatoes wedges in the tray. Flatten it well to make one layer.
- Preheat the oven to 375F.
- Place the tray with potatoes in the oven and bake for 40 minutes. Stir the potatoes from time to time.
- The potato fries are cooked when they have crunchy edges.

Nutrition: calories 122, fat 11.6, fiber 0.5, carbs 4.5, protein 0.6

Lemon Cauliflower Florets

Preparation Time: 15 minutes

Cooking Time: 12 minutes

Servings:6

Ingredients:

1-pound cauliflower head, trimmed

3 tablespoons lemon juice

3 eggs, beaten

1 teaspoon salt

1 teaspoon ground black pepper

2 cups water, for cooking

3 tablespoons almond butter

1 teaspoon turmeric

Directions:

Place the cauliflower head in the pan.

- Add water.

- Boil the cauliflower for 8 minutes or until tender.

- Cool the vegetable well and separate into florets.

- Whisk together the beaten eggs, salt, ground black pepper, and turmeric.

- Dip each cauliflower floret in the egg mixture.

- Toss the almond butter in the skillet and heat up.

- Roast the cauliflower florets for 2 minutes on each side over the medium heat.

- When the cauliflower florets are golden brown, they are done.

- Sprinkle the cooked florets with lemon juice.

Nutrition: calories 103, fat 6.9, fiber 2.9, carbs 6.3, protein 6.1

Chapter 6:
Desserts

Poached Cherries

Preparation Time: 10 minutes

Cooking Time: 10 minutes

Servings: 5(1/2 cup each)

Ingredients:

1 pound fresh and sweet cherries, rinsed, pitted

3 strips (1x3 inches each) orange zest,

3 strips (1x3 inches each) lemon zest,

2/3 cup sugar

15 peppercorns

1/4 vanilla bean, split but not scraped

1 3/4 cups water

Directions:

- In a saucepan, mix the water, citrus zest, sugar, peppercorns, and vanilla bean; bring to a boil, stirring until the sugar is dissolved.

- Add the cherries; simmer for about 10 minutes until the cherries are soft, but not falling apart.

- Skim any foam from the surface and let the poached cherries cool.

- Refrigerate with the poaching liquid. Before serving, strain the cherries.

Nutrition: 170 Calories, 1 g total fat (0 g sat. fat, 0 g mono fat, 0.5 g poly fat), 0 mg Chol., 0 mg sodium, 42 g total carbs., and 2 g fiber.

Watermelon-Strawberry Rosewater Yogurt Panna Cotta

Preparation Time: 20 minutes

Cooking Time: 5 minutes

Servings: 4

Ingredients:

500 g seedless watermelon, peeled, and cut into 5-mm pieces

3 teaspoons rosewater

250 ml honey-flavored yogurt

250 ml (1 cup) thickened cream

2 teaspoons gelatin powder

2 tablespoons caster sugar

10 strawberries, washed, hulled, and cut into 5-mm pieces

1 tablespoon hot water

honey, to serve

vegetable oil, to grease

Directions:

- Brush 4 pieces of 125 ml or 1/2 cup sprinkle molds with vegetable oil to grease.

- Put the yogurt into a large-sized heat-safe bowl.

- Place the sugar and cream into a small-sized saucepan and heat over medium heat; stir until the sugar is heated through and dissolved.

- Place the hot water into a small-sized heat-safe bowl. Sprinkle the gelatin over the hot water. Place the bowl into a small-sized saucepan.

- Add enough boiling water to fill the saucepan about 3/4 deep on the side of the bowl. With a fork, whisk the mixture until the gelatin is dissolved.

- Add the gelatin and cream mixture into the yogurt, whisking until well combined. Strain the mixture through a fine sieve over a large-sized jug.

- Pour the strained mixture into the prepared molds. Cover each mold with a plastic wrap.

- Refrigerate for at least 6 hours or overnight until set.

- In a medium bowl, combine the strawberry, watermelon, and rosewater.

- Turn the panna cottas into serving bowl. Spoon the strawberry-watermelon over each panna cotta.

- Drizzle with honey and serve.

Notes: for a different version, omit the rosewater, strawberries, and honey. Combine the watermelon with 1/3 cup of fresh passion fruit pulp, and spoon over the panna cotta.

Nutrition: 364.96 Calories, 26 g total fat (16 g sat. fat), 75 mg Chol., 69.54 mg sodium, 26 g total carbs., 26 g sugar, 7 g protein, and 1 g fiber.

Mascarpone and Ricotta Stuffed Dates

Preparation Time: 20 minutes

Cooking Time: 10 minutes

Servings: 5

Ingredients:

125 g fresh ricotta

125 g mascarpone

2 teaspoons finely grated orange rind

30 pieces fresh dates

45 g (1/4 cup) dry roasted hazelnuts, coarsely chopped, for sprinkling

45 g (1/4 cup) icing sugar mixture

For the Frangelico syrup:

80 ml (1/3 cup) Frangelico liqueur

125 ml (1/2 cup) water

215 g (1 cup) caster sugar

Directions:

- Beat the mascarpone, icing sugar, ricotta, and orange rind in a large-sized bowl until mixture is smooth.

- With a sharp knife, cut a slit in each date. Remove the pits and discard. Spoon 1 heaped teaspoon of the ricotta mixture into each date.

To make the Frangelico syrup:

- Put the water and the sugar into a medium-sized saucepan. Heat over low heat; cook for about 2 to 3 minutes, stirring until the sugar is dissolved. Increase the heat to high and bring the mixture to a boil.

- Cook for 5 minutes without stirring or until the syrup is slightly thick. Stir the Frangelico liqueur. Remove from saucepan from the heat, set aside for 30 minutes to cool.

- Put the dates on a serving platter. Pour the Frangelico syrup over the dates. Sprinkle with hazelnuts and serve.

Nutrition: 115.92 Calories, 3.5 g total fat (1.5 g sat. fat), 26 g total carbs., 20 g sugar, 1.5 g protein, and 1 g fiber.

Glazed Mediterranean Puffy Fig

Preparation Time: 5 minutes

Cooking Time: 25 minutes

Servings: 8

Ingredients:

2 sheets (from 1 pack of 4 sheets) puff pastry

20 figs or dry figs (dry or fresh)

8 ounces mascarpone cheese

2 tablespoons butter

1/2 cup (or 8 tablespoons) honey

1/2 teaspoon cinnamon

1/2 teaspoon nutmeg

1/4 teaspoon salt

4 mint leaves, for garnish

Directions:

- Preheat the oven 400F.

- Slice puff pastry into triangle and place into a nonstick baking sheet; bake for about 15-20 minutes or until golden brown. When baked, remove from the oven and allow to cool.

- If using dry figs, rehydrate for 1 hour and then cut into half. Put the butter into a nonstick pan over medium flame or heat.

- Add the figs; cook for about 3 to 5 minutes. Add the honey, salt, cinnamon, and nutmeg; cook, stirring, for about 3 minutes.

- Remove the skillet from hat and allow to cool for about 5 to 10 minutes.

- Place a pastry slice on a plate, top with 1 tablespoon of cheese, some figs, and then drizzle with the glaze. Repeat the topping, if desired. Garnish with mint leaves and serve.

Nutrition: 486 Calories, 22.8 g total fat (8.3 g sat. fat), 22 mg Chol., 226 mg sodium, 391 mg pot., 67.4 g total carbs., 5.4 g fiber, 40.6 g sugar, 7.9 g protein

Figs Pie

Preparation Time: 10 minutes

Cooking Time: 1 hour

Servings: 8

Ingredients:

½ cup stevia

6 figs, cut into quarters

½ teaspoon vanilla extract

1 cup almond flour

4 eggs, whisked

Directions:

- Spread the figs on the bottom of a springform pan lined with parchment paper.
- In a bowl, combine the other ingredients, whisk and pour over the figs.
- Bake at 375 digress F for 1 hour, flip the pie upside down when done and serve.

Nutrition: calories 200, fat 4.4, fiber 3, carbs 7.6, protein 8

Cherry Cream

Preparation Time: 2 hours

Cooking Time: 0 minutes

Servings: 4

Ingredients:

2 cups cherries, pitted and chopped

1 cup almond milk

½ cup whipping cream

3 eggs, whisked

1/3 cup Stevia

1 teaspoon lemon juice

½ teaspoon vanilla extract

Directions:

- In your food processor, combine cherries with the milk and the rest of the ingredients.
- Pulse well, divide into cups and keep in the fridge for 2 hours before serving.

Nutrition: calories 200, fat 4.5, fiber 3.3, carbs 5.6, protein 3.4

Strawberries Cream

Preparation Time: 10 minutes

Cooking Time: 20 minutes

Servings: 4

Ingredients:

½ cup stevia

2 pounds strawberries, chopped

1 cup almond milk

zest of 1 lemon, grated

½ cup heavy cream

3 egg yolks, whisked

Directions:

- Heat a pan with the milk over medium-high heat, add the Stevia and the rest of the ingredients, whisk well.
- Simmer for 20 minutes, divide into cups and serve cold.

Nutrition: calories 152, fat 4.4, fiber 5.5, carbs 5.1, protein 0.8

Apples and Plum Cake

Preparation Time: 10 minutes

Cooking Time: 40 minutes

Servings: 4

Ingredients:

7 ounces almond flour

1 egg, whisked

5 tablespoons Stevia

3 ounces warm almond milk

2 pounds plums, pitted and cut into quarters

2 apples, cored and chopped

zest of 1 lemon

1 teaspoon baking powder

Directions:

- In a bowl, mix the almond milk with the egg, Stevia, and the rest of the ingredients except the cooking spray and whisk well.
- Grease a cake pan with the oil, pour the cake mix inside, Place in the oven and bake at 350 degrees F for 40 minutes.
- Cool, slice and serve.

Nutrition: calories 209, fat 6.4, fiber 6, carbs 8, protein 6.6

Cinnamon Chickpeas Cookies

Preparation Time: 10 minutes

Cooking Time: 20 minutes

Servings: 12

Ingredients:

1 cup canned chickpeas, drained, rinsed and mashed

2 cups almond flour

1 teaspoon cinnamon powder

1 teaspoon baking powder

1 cup avocado oil

½ cup Stevia

1 egg, whisked

2 teaspoons almond extract

1 cup raisins

1 cup coconut, unsweetened and shredded

Directions:

- In a bowl, combine the chickpeas with the flour, cinnamon and other ingredients, and whisk well until you obtain a dough.
- Scoop tablespoons of dough on a baking sheet lined with parchment paper, Place them in the oven at 350 degrees F and bake for 20 minutes.
- Let them cool down for a few minutes and serve.

Nutrition: calories 200, fat 4.5, fiber 3.4, carbs 9.5, protein 2.4

Cocoa Brownies

Preparation Time: 10 minutes

Cooking Time: 20 minutes

Servings: 8

Ingredients:

30 ounces canned lentils, rinsed and drained

1 tablespoon honey

1 banana, peeled and chopped

½ teaspoon baking soda

4 tablespoons almond butter

2 tablespoons cocoa powder

cooking spray

Directions:

- In a food processor, combine the lentils with the honey and the other ingredients except the cooking spray and pulse well.

- Pour this into a pan greased with cooking spray, spread evenly, Place in the oven at 375 degrees F and bake for 20 minutes.

- Cut the brownies and serve cold.

Nutrition: calories 200, fat 4.5, fiber 2.4 carbs 8.7, protein 4.3

Cranberries and Pears Pie

Preparation Time: 10 minutes

Cooking Time: 40 minutes

Servings: 4

Ingredients:

2 cup cranberries

3 cups pears, cubed

A drizzle of olive oil

1 cup Stevia

1/3 cup almond flour

1 cup rolled oats

¼ avocado oil

Directions:

- In a bowl, mix the cranberries with the pears and other ingredients except the olive oil and oats, and stir well.

- Grease a cake pan with a drizzle of olive oil, pour the pear mix inside, sprinkle the oats all over and bake at 350 degrees F for 40 minutes.

- Cool mix down and serve.

Nutrition: calories 172, fat 3.4, fiber 4.3, carbs 11.5, protein 4.5

Lemon Cream

Preparation Time: 1 hour

Cooking Time: 10 minutes

Servings: 6

Ingredients:

2 eggs, whisked

1 and ¼ cup Stevia

10 tablespoons avocado oil

1 cup heavy cream

Juice of 2 lemons

Zest of 2 lemons, grated

Directions:

- In a pan, combine the cream with the lemon juice and other ingredients, whisk well, cook for 10 minutes.
- Divide into cups and keep in the fridge for 1 hour before serving.

Nutrition: calories 200, fat 8.5, fiber 4.5, carbs 8.6, protein 4.5

Blueberries Stew

Preparation Time: 10 minutes

Cooking Time: 10 minutes

Servings: 4

Ingredients:

2 cups blueberries

3 tablespoons Stevia

1 and ½ cups pure apple juice

1 teaspoon vanilla extract

Directions:

- In a pan, combine the blueberries with Stevia and other ingredients, bring to a simmer and cook over medium-low heat for 10 minutes.
- Divide into cups and serve cold.

Nutrition: calories 192, fat 5.4, fiber 3.4, carbs 9.4, protein 4.5

Mandarin Cream

Preparation Time: 20 minutes

Cooking Time: 0 minutes

Servings: 8

Ingredients:

2 mandarins, peeled and cut into segments

Juice of 2 mandarins

2 tablespoons stevia

4 eggs, whisked

¾ cup stevia

¾ cup almonds, ground

Directions:

- In a blender, combine the mandarins with the mandarins juice and the other ingredients, whisk well.
- Divide into cups and keep in the fridge for 20 minutes before serving.

Nutrition: calories 106, fat 3.4, fiber 0, carbs 2.4, protein 4

Creamy Mint Strawberry Mix

Preparation Time: 10 minutes

Cooking Time: 30 minutes

Servings: 6

Ingredients:

cooking spray

¼ cup stevia

1 and ½ cup almond flour

1 teaspoon baking powder

1 cup almond milk

1 egg, whisked

2 cups strawberries, sliced

1 tablespoon mint, chopped

1 teaspoon lime zest, grated

½ cup whipping cream

Directions:

- In a bowl, combine the almond with the strawberries, mint and the other ingredients except the cooking spray and whisk well.
- Grease 6 ramekins with the cooking spray, pour the strawberry mix inside,
- Place in the oven and bake at 350 degrees F for 30 minutes.
- Cool and serve.

Nutrition: calories 200, fat 6.3, fiber 2, carbs 6.5, protein 8

Vanilla Cake

Preparation Time: 10 minutes

Cooking Time: 25 minutes

Servings: 10

Ingredients:

3 cups almond flour

3 teaspoons baking powder

1 cup olive oil

1 and ½ cup almond milk

1 and 2/3 cup stevia

2 cups water

1 tablespoon lime juice

2 teaspoons vanilla extract

cooking spray

Directions:

- In a bowl, mix the almond flour with the baking powder, the oil and the rest of the ingredients except the cooking spray and whisk well.
- Pour mix into a cake pan greased with cooking spray, Place in the oven and bake at 370 degrees F for 25 minutes.
- Leave the cake to cool down, cut and serve!

Nutrition: calories 200, fat 7.6, fiber 2.5, carbs 5.5, protein 4.5

Pumpkin Cream

Preparation Time: 5 minutes

Cooking Time: 5 minutes

Servings: 2

Ingredients:

2 cups canned pumpkin flesh

2 tablespoons stevia

1 teaspoon vanilla extract

2 tablespoons water

pinch of pumpkin spice

Directions:

- In a pan, combine the pumpkin flesh with the other ingredients, simmer for 5 minutes.

- Divide into cups and serve cold.

Nutrition: calories 192, fat 3.4, fiber 4.5, carbs 7.6, protein 3.5

Grapes Stew

Preparation Time: 10 minutes

Cooking Time: 10 minutes

Servings: 4

Ingredients:

2/3 cup Stevia

1 tablespoon olive oil

1/3 cup coconut water

1 teaspoon vanilla extract

1 teaspoon lemon zest, grated

2 cup red grapes, halved

Directions:

- Heat a pan with the water over medium heat, add oil, Stevia and the rest of the ingredients.

- Toss, simmer for 10 minutes, divide into cups, and serve.

Nutrition: calories 122, fat 3.7, fiber 1.2, carbs 2.3, protein 0.4

Cocoa Sweet Cherry Cream

Preparation Time: 2 hours

Cooking Time: 0 minutes

Servings: 4

Ingredients:

½ cup cocoa powder

¾ cup red cherry jam

¼ cup stevia

2 cups water

1 pound cherries, pitted and halved

Directions:

- In a blender, mix the cherries with the water and the rest of the ingredients, pulse well.
- Divide into cups and keep in the fridge for 2 hours before serving.

Nutrition: calories 162, fat 3.4, fiber 2.4, carbs 5, protein 1

Apple Couscous Pudding

Preparation Time: 10 minutes

Cooking Time: 25 minutes

Servings: 4

Ingredients:

½ cup couscous

1 and ½ cups milk

¼ cup apple, cored and chopped

3 tablespoons stevia

½ teaspoon rose water

1 tablespoon orange zest, grated

Directions:

- Heat a pan with the milk over medium heat, add the couscous and the rest of the ingredients, whisk, simmer for 25 minutes.
- Divide into bowls and serve.

Nutrition: calories 150, fat 4.5, fiber 5.5, carbs 7.5, protein 4

Ricotta Ramekins

Preparation Time: 10 minutes

Cooking Time: 1 hour

Servings: 4

Ingredients:

6 eggs, whisked

1 and ½ pounds ricotta cheese, soft

½ pound stevia

1 teaspoon vanilla extract

½ teaspoon baking powder

cooking spray

Directions:

- In a bowl, mix the eggs with the ricotta and the other ingredients except the cooking spray and whisk well.
- Grease 4 ramekins with the cooking spray, pour the ricotta cream in each and bake at 360 degrees F for 1 hour.
- Serve cold.

Nutrition: calories 180, fat 5.3, fiber 5.4, carbs 11.5, protein 4

Papaya Cream

Preparation Time: 10 minutes

Cooking Time: 0 minutes

Servings: 2

Ingredients:

1 cup papaya, peeled and chopped

1 cup heavy cream

1 tablespoon Stevia

½ teaspoon vanilla extract

Directions:

- In a blender, combine the cream with the papaya and the other ingredients, pulse well.

- Divide into cups and serve cold.

Nutrition: calories 182, fat 3.1, fiber 2.3, carbs 3.5, protein 2

Mediterranean Stuffed Custard Pancakes

Preparation Time: 60 minutes

Cooking Time: 20 minutes

Servings: 10

Ingredients:

For the batter:

2 cups flour

1/2 cup whole-wheat flour

2 cups milk

1 cup water

1 teaspoon yeast

1 teaspoon baking powder

1 teaspoon sugar

For the custard:

2 cups whole milk

2 cups fat-free milk or 2 % milk

1 cup heavy cream

3 tablespoons sugar

1/2 cup cornstarch

1/2 cup water

7 pieces medium-sized white bread, crust removed

1 tablespoon rose water

1 tablespoon orange blossom water

For the topping:

1 cup pistachio

1 tablespoon honey or simple syrup

Directions:

For the custard:

- In a medium-sized pot, pour in the milks, heavy cream, cornstarch, and sugar; heat the mixture, stirring.

- Cut the bread into pieces and add into the pot; stir until the mixture starts to thicken.

- Add the orange and rose water; stir until the custard is very thick. Remove from the heat and then pour into a bowl; let cool for 1 hour, stirring every 15 minutes.

- Cover with Saran wrap and then refrigerate to completely cool.

For the batter:

- Mix all the batter ingredients in a mixing bowl, stirring until well combined; let sit for 20 minutes.

- Over medium-low flame or heat, heat a nonstick pan. Pour 1/4 cup-worth of the batter to make a 3-inch diameter pancake; cook for about 30 seconds or until the top of the batter is bubbly and no longer wet and the bottom is golden brown.

- Transfer into a dish to cool. Repeat the process with the remaining batter.

To assemble:

- Take out the bowl of custard from the refrigerator. Transfer the chilled custard into a piping bag.

- Fold a pancake together, pinching the edges to make a pocket. Pipe the custard into the pancake pocket, filling it.

- Repeat the process with the remaining pancakes and custard. Top each filled pocket with the ground pistachio. Refrigerate until ready to serve.

- To serve, transfer the custard-filled pancakes into a Servings plate; drizzle with honey or simple syrup.

Nutrition: 450 Calories, 19 g total fat (8 g sat. fat), 42.9 mg Chol., 241.5 mg sodium, 60 g total carbs., 2.8 g fiber, 16.6 g sugar, 13 g protein, 10.3% vitamin A, 2% vitamin C, 31.2% calcium, and 11.5% iron.

Mediterranean Cheesecake

Preparation Time: 15 minutes

Cooking Time: 20 minutes

Servings: 8

Ingredients:

1 package (8 ounces) cream cheese

1/4 cup sour cream

1/2 cup condensed milk, sweetened

5 tablespoons sugar, divided

1 tablespoon vanilla

1 tablespoon orange blossom

1 tablespoon rose water

1 tablespoon orange zest

1 egg

1/2 cup butter

2 cups phyllo dough or kadaifi

1/2 cup toasted coconut

1/2 cup pistachios

1/2 cup simple syrup

Directions:

Preheat the oven to 325F.

- With a hand mixer, mix the condensed milk, cream cheese, and the sour cream in a large bowl until well blended.

- Add the orange zest, orange blossom, rose water, vanilla, and sugar, blend for 1 minute. Add in the egg and blend for 30 seconds.

- In another bowl, break the kadaifi into pieces. Add 3 tablespoons of the sugar and the butter, mix until well combined.

- Line the bottom and the sides of a cheesecake pan or a muffin tin with the kadaifi mixture.

- Pour the cheesecake mixture into the cheesecake pan or muffin tin, filling 80% of the container. Place into the oven and bake for 20 minutes. Remove from the oven and let completely cool before Servings.

- When completely cool, slice the cake into 8 portions, top with the syrup, pistachio and/or coconut, and glaze with more simple syrup. Serve.

Nutrition: 742 Calories, 43 g total fat (23 g sat. fat), 129.3 mg Chol., 526.5 mg sodium, 78 g total carbs., 2.6 g fiber, 43.1 g sugar, 12 g protein

Mediterranean Bread Pudding

Preparation Time: 10 minutes, plus 6 hr. chilling

Cooking Time: 20 minutes

Servings: 6

Ingredients:

1/4 of a large-sized lemon, juiced

1/2 cup sugar

8 white bread slices, edges removed, toasted, or more as needed

2 cups Ashta or Lebanese cream, or more as needed

1 1/2 cup simple syrup

1/2 cup shredded coconut, toasted

1/2 cup pine nuts

Directions:

- Put the sugar, lemon juice, and water into a thick-bottomed pan. Place the pan on the stove and heat over high flame or heat; bring to a boil, continuously stirring.

- When boiling, let it simmer for 5 minutes, continuously stirring, until the mixture is amber in color, being careful it does not burn and turn bitter.

- Choose a metal pan according to your desired size. Immediately pour the caramel into the pan, swirling the pan to spread the caramel evenly.

- In a single layer, arrange the toasted bread on top of the caramel layer. Generously pour the simple syrup over the bread and spread with the Ashta.

- If you are using a small metal pan, repeat the layer of bread, drizzle of caramel, and Ashta. Generously sprinkle with the coconut and the pine nuts.

- Cover the pan and refrigerate for at least 6 hours or overnight. When chilled, slice into 6 portion sand serve.

Notes: you can decorate this dessert with your preferred choice of topping, such as pistachios, almonds, strawberries, candied orange, etc. You can even layer the ingredients in glasses or ramekins for a fancy presentation.

Nutrition: 619 Calories, 10 g total fat (2.6 g sat. fat), 0 mg Chol., 208.3 mg sodium, 130 g total carbs., 5.3 g fiber, 94.6 g sugar, 5 g protein

Banana Shake Bowls

Preparation Time: 5 minutes

Cooking Time: 0 minutes

Servings: 4

Ingredients:

4 medium bananas, peeled

1 avocado, peeled, pitted and mashed

¾ cup almond milk

½ teaspoon vanilla extract

Directions:

- In a blender, combine the bananas with the avocado and other ingredients, pulse.
- Divide into bowls and keep in the fridge until serving.

Nutrition: calories 185, fat 4.3, fiber 4, carbs 6, protein 6.45

Mediterranean Biscotti

Preparation Time: 25 minutes

Cooking Time: 1 hour

Servings: 3 dozen

Ingredients:

2 eggs

1 cup whole-wheat flour

1 cup all-purpose flour

3/4 cup Parmesan cheese, grated

2 teaspoons baking powder

2 tablespoons sugar

1/4 cup sun-dried tomato, finely chopped

1/4 cup Kalamata olive, finely chopped

1/3 cup olive oil

1/2 teaspoon salt

1/2 teaspoon black pepper, cracked

1 teaspoon dried oregano (preferably Greek)

1 teaspoon dried basil

Directions:

- Into a large-sized bowl, beat the eggs and the sugar together. Pour in the olive; beat until smooth.

- In another bowl, combine the flours, baking powder, pepper, salt, oregano, and basil. Stir the flour mix into the egg mixture, stirring until blended.

- Stir in the cheese, tomatoes, and olives; stirring until thoroughly combined.

- Divide the dough into 2 portions; shape each into 10-inch long logs. Place the logs into a parchment-lined cookie sheet; flatten the log tops slightly.

- Bake for about 30 minutes in a preheated 375F oven or until the logs are pale golden and not quite firm to the touch.

- Remove from the oven; let cool on the baking sheet for 3 minutes. Transfer the logs into a cutting board; slice each log into 1/2-inch diagonal slices using a serrated knife.

- Place the biscotti slices on the baking sheet, return into the 325F oven, and bake for about 20 to 25 minutes until dry and firm.

- Flip the slices halfway through baking. Remove from the oven, transfer on a wire rack and let cool.

Notes: store the biscotti in airtight containers.

Nutrition: 731.6 Calories, 36.5 g total fat (9 g sat. fat), 146 mg Chol., 1238.4 mg sodium, 77.8 g carb., 3.5 g fiber, 10.7 g sugar, and 23.3 g protein.

Chocolate Baklava

Preparation Time: 46 minutes

Cooking Time: 35 minutes

Servings: 24(1 piece)

Ingredients:

24 sheets (14 x 9-inch) frozen whole-wheat phyllo (filo) dough, thawed

1/8 teaspoon salt

1/3 cup toasted walnuts, chopped coarsely

1/3 cup almonds, blanched toasted, chopped coarsely

1/2 teaspoon ground cinnamon

1/2 cup water

1/2 cup hazelnuts, toasted, chopped coarsely

1/2 cup pistachios, roasted, chopped coarsely

3/4 cup honey

1/2 cup of butter, melted

1 cup chocolate-hazelnut spread (like Nutella)

1-piece (3-inch) cinnamon stick

cooking spray

Directions:

- In a medium-sized saucepan, combine the water, honey, and the cinnamon stick; stir until the honey is dissolved.

- Increase the heat/flame to medium; continue cooking for about 10 minutes without stirring. The candy thermometer should read 230F.

- Remove the saucepan from the heat and then keep warm. Remove and discard the cinnamon stick.

- Preheat the oven to 350F.

- Put the chocolate-hazelnut spread into microwavable bowl; microwave the spread for about 30 seconds on HIGH or until the spread is melted.

- In a bowl, combine the hazelnuts, pistachios, almonds, walnuts, ground cinnamon, and the salt.

- Lightly grease with the cooking spray a 9x13-inch ceramic or glass baking dish.

- Put 1 sheet lengthwise into the bottom of the prepared baking dish, extending the ends of the sheet over the edges of the dish.

- Lightly brush the sheet with the butter. Repeat the process with 5 sheets phyllo and a light brush of butter.

- Drizzle 1/3 cup of the melted chocolate-hazelnut spread over the buttered phyllo sheets. Sprinkle about 1/3 of the nut mixture (1/2 cup) over the spread.

- Repeat the process, layering phyllo sheet, brush of butter, spread, and with nut mixture. For the last, nut mixture top layer, top with 6 phyllo sheets, pressing each phyllo gently into the dish and brushing each sheet with butter.

- Slice the layers into 24 portions by making 3 cuts lengthwise and then 5 cuts crosswise with a sharp knife; bake for about 35 minutes at 350F or until the phyllo sheets are golden.

- Remove the dish from the oven, drizzle the honey sauce over the baklava. Pace the dish on a wire rack and let cool.

- Cover and store the baklava at normal room temperature if not serve right away.

Nutrition: 238 Calories, 13.4 g total fat (4.3 g sat. fat, 5.6 g mono fat, 2 g poly fat), 4 g protein, 27.8 g total carbs., 1.6 g fiber, 10 mg

Orange-Glazed Fruit and Ouzo Whipped Cream

Preparation Time: 20 minutes, plus 30 minutes chilling

Cooking Time: 10 minutes

Servings: 4

Ingredients:

3 cups fruit (such as tangerine wedges, quartered apricots or plums, or strips of mango)

1 tablespoon olive oil spread/butter divided (I Can't Believe It's Not Butter! ®), melted

chopped almonds, optional (or pistachios)

For the ouzo whipped cream:

1 teaspoon sugar

1 teaspoon ouzo liqueur (anise-flavored), orange juice, orange liqueur, or several drops of anise extract

1/2 cup whipping cream

For the sauce:

2 tablespoons sugar

2 tablespoons honey

1/4 cup orange juice

Directions:

For the syrup:

- Mix the syrup ingredients inside a small-sized saucepan. Bring the mixture to a boil, stirring, until the honey and the sugar are dissolved and reduce the heat.

- Simmer the mixture, without cover, for 10 minutes and set aside.

For the ouzo whipped cream:

- In a medium-sized chilled bowl, beat the ouzo whipped cream ingredients using electric mixer on medium speed until soft peaks form with the tips curled.

- Cover and refrigerate for about 30 minutes to chill.

For the grilled fruit:

- Toss the melted olive oil butter and fruit in a mixing bowl. Transfer the fruit to a foil or grill pan.

- If using a charcoal grill, put pan with fruits on an uncovered grill rack over medium coals; grill for about 10-12 minutes, stirring occasionally, until fruits are heated through.

- If using a gas grill, first preheat the grill, then reduce to medium heat. Put the grill rack on the grill rack. Cover and grill for about 10-12 minutes, stirring occasionally, until the fruits are heated through.

- Divide the fruits between 4 pieces dessert plates and drizzle with the honey syrup. If desired, sprinkle with the almonds. Serve with the ouzo whipped cream.

Nutrition: 267 Calories, 15 g total fat, 44 mg sodium, 49 mg Chol., 36 g total carbs., 26 g sugar, 2 g fiber, and 2 g protein.

Conclusion

The Mediterranean way of eating is one of the most popular and beloved eating patterns around, known for its health benefits and slimming properties. This tasty diet is based on fresh, plant-based foods that are rich in healthy fats as well as whole foods that grow from the ground.

People who live in the Mediterranean region (Italy, Balkans, Spain, Portugal, France) are known to have fit figures, live longer, and in general, are healthy. This is a diet (or an eating pattern) with no strict rules. All it suggests is you get the right ingredients such as fruits, vegetables, olive oil, fish, and seafood, and do what works the best for you.

If your main goal is to lose weight while eating Mediterranean meals, then you will make a wonderful choice. Slimming with this diet goes steadily and in a healthy way. There is no restriction or starvation, but rather eating foods that are not processed.

Switching to the fresh and whole foods might be challenging if you are used to eating fast food, red and processed meats, sweets, white flour, sugar, and alcohol.

The risk of cancer, heart failures, high blood pressure, cholesterol, depression, inflammations, poor immunity, and other health issues is significantly higher when your menu consists mostly of unhealthy food. This should serve as ample motivation.

This diet is a sure way to purge your blood, improve your general mood and health, boost your immunity, and lower the risk of evil diseases such as type 2 diabetes, breast and colon cancer, or Alzheimer's disease.

Studies have shown that even depression and anxiety are directly connected with one's choice of food. Foods that grew naturally and under the sun have a far bigger chance of improving your mood and boosting your body serotonin. One of the greatest things about the Mediterranean way of eating is that you do not have to be an extraordinary cook to prepare your meals. With the right ingredients, you can always make simple and delicious meals that don't require hours in the kitchen. The recipes provided are clear proof!

Prepare your weekly meal plan, buy the groceries, and simply stick to eating suitable foods. Your energy will be higher, your brain's cognitive functions and memory will improve, and you will never feel bloated. Digestion will become easier, and you will feel happier.

The most important thing for people who want to slim down with this diet is to keep a positive mindset. This is a healthy lifestyle that requires you to pay attention to the food you are eating, spend more time with your loved ones, and do more physical activity. Once you lose weight, you will maintain your figure by simply eating your favorite meals. Since this diet does not feel like a diet, it is super easy for following.

There is no yo-yo effect because you will remain true to the prescribed Mediterranean menu. This diet is a wonderful way to get rid of unhealthy eating habits and kill all those cravings for junk food. At the end of the day, nothing is forbidden in this diet. Certain foods are recommended to be consumed frequently, while others should be eaten every once in a while.

When you see that you have lost a couple of pounds within the first week, you will know that you made the right decision. Finally, what matters is that you feel content, happy, and good in your skin. I hope this book answered most of your questions and helped you make a decision to start your new lifestyle.

www.ingramcontent.com/pod-product-compliance
Lightning Source LLC
Chambersburg PA
CBHW061504050726
47593CB00002B/452